© 2015 Viva-eBooks All rights reserved. No part of this book may be reproduced or transferred in any form or by any means, graphic, electronic or mechanical, including photocopying, scanning, recording, taping or by any other information storage retrieval system with the express written permission of the author. Any trademarks that are used are used without any consent and the publication of the trademark is without permission or backing by the trademark owner. All trademarks and brands within this book are for ... ... ir respective owners and not affiliated with this document. V ... ... ador mentioned in this book. The fact that an individual, organi ... ... tion and/or potential source of further information does not m ... ... ation the individual, organisation or website may provide or rec ...

This book is sold on the understanding that the publisher ... ... gal or other professional advice or services. The information pro ... ... ou require professional or medical advice or treatment for a s ... ... fied professional person should be sought promptly. Achieving and maintaining a healthy weight is an ambition that would benefit most overweight adults and following a diet plan can help achieve this. However, the 5:2 diet plan is not suitable for:

- anyone who is pregnant, planning a pregnancy or breast-feeding
- anyone with a major health condition such as diabetes, irritable bowel syndrome
- anyone who has had an eating disorder.

In any case, you should consult your doctor before commencing a new diet or exercise regime.

This book is designed to provide general information in regard to the subject matter. While reasonable attempts have been made to verify the accuracy of the information provided, neither the author nor the publisher assumes any responsibility for errors, omissions, interpretations or usage of the subject matters within.

Warning on Allergic reactions –some recipes included in this book use nuts or nut oils. These specific recipes should be avoided by:

- anyone with a known nut allergy
- anyone who may be vulnerable to nut allergies such as pregnant and nursing mothers, invalids, the elderly, babies and children.

Warning on Eggs –The UK Department of Health's advice is that eggs should not be consumed raw. Some recipes included in this book are made with raw or lightly cooked eggs. These specific recipes should be avoided by:

- anyone who may be vulnerable such as pregnant and nursing mothers, invalids, the elderly, babies and children.

MillyWhiteCooks.com

facebook.com/MillyWhiteCooks

pinterest.com/MillyWhiteCooks

instagram.com/MillyWhiteCooks

twitter.com/MillyWhiteCooks

plus.google.com/+MillywhitecooksBooks/posts

CONTENTS

INTRODUCTION TO THE TWO-DAY 5:2 DIET PLAN — 3
  The Basic Principles — 5

DIET FOR TWO DAYS, FEAST FOR FIVE — 6
  The Easy Three Steps to the Two-day 5:2 Diet Plan — 6

HOW TO USE THIS RECIPE COOKBOOK — 9

HELPFUL TIPS AND TRICKS FOR THE TWO-DAY 5:2 DIET PLAN — 10

EXAMPLE DAY MENU PLANNERS — 12
  500 calorie Example Menu Plans — 12
  600 calorie Example Menu Plans — 13

TWO-DAY 5:2 DIET BREAKFASTS — 14
  100 Calories & Under — 14
  150 Calories & Under — 17
  200 Calories & Under — 20

TWO-DAY 5:2 DIET LUNCHES — 23
  150 Calories & Under — 23
  200 Calories & Under — 29

TWO-DAY 5:2 DIET DINNERS — 34
  200 Calories & Under — 34
  300 Calories & Under — 44

A NOTE FROM THE AUTHOR — 56
  Further Two-day 5:2 Diet Books — 56
  Your Bonus 5:2 Diet Plan Free Giveaway — 56
  Let's Stay Connected — 57

INDEX — 58

INTRODUCTION

THE TWO-DAY 5:2 DIET PLAN – THE BASIC PRINCIPLES

Are you intrigued by a diet plan which offers an effective solution that will help you lose weight and improve your health, whilst still allowing you to eat all of the foods that you love? What about a diet plan that allows you to be relaxed and free to eat well on five days a week? Does this sound to good to be true? Have you previously started a new diet plan only to end up feeling let down, discouraged and defeated?

If you are reading this cookbook, it is likely that you are already familiar with the concept of the 5:2 Diet, sometimes referred to as Intermittent Fasting. In some cultures and religions, intermittent fasting has been practised for hundreds of years. More recently, following a UK documentary programme first broadcast in 2012, it has become one of the most popular and widely followed diet regimes. This book will explain:

- why the Two-Day 5:2 Diet Plan has become so popular
- whether following the Two-Day 5:2 Diet Plan can lead to weight loss
- whether the Two-Day 5:2 Diet Plan is a healthy diet plan and suitable for anyone
- what to eat on the diet days on the Two-Day 5:2 Diet Plan
- eating well on your 5 non-diet days
- the easy three-steps to the Two-Day 5:2 Diet Plan
- 5 top tips for stress-free diet days
- 7 really useful diet day bits of kitchen kit.

As well as providing all the information that you need to start following the 5 Two-Day 5:2 Diet Plan, you will find a delicious selection of easy, tasty recipes to help make your diet days successful.

WHY IS THE TWO-DAY 5:2 DIET PLAN IS SO POPULAR?

There are a number for reasons for this. Firstly, it is **a simple concept** that is extremely easy to follow, as you just diet on a two days a week and then eat normally (but healthily) on the remaining 5 days.

This means that it is **a very convenient diet plan** to follow even if you normally struggle to incorporate dieting into your lifestyle, perhaps because you work shifts, or travel on business, for example?

The 5:2 diet also **suits anyone who has struggled to maintain their will-power** or **become very bored of the routine when dieting** over a sustained period of time. With the 5:2 diet plan, as you diet for just two (non-consecutive) days a week, you:

- only need to maintain will-power in short bursts
- don't get bored as within 24 hrs you can eat whatever tickles your taste buds!

ARE YOU A YO-YO DIETER?

Before I cover how the 5:2 Diet plan works, I would like to specifically address anyone who has tried and failed to diet before, especially if you have previously been a "yo-yo" dieter. By this I mean that you've started a diet with great intentions and the will-power of a saint, but after a period of time (and that may be a week, a month, 6 months), suddenly you've faltered and that falter has resulted in a binge. Often this is because a diet is about restrictions and forbidden items, and you need to keep to that regime day-in, day out, week-in, week-out. We are all human, and often we eat for reasons that are more than just to give us the energy we need to exist. We eat to celebrate and to commiserate, we eat out of boredom, we eat out of joy, we eat to be social and many more reasons besides.

If you have been through the cycle of yo-yo dieting previously, the Two-Day 5:2 Diet Plan is the antithesis of this. It could be argued that it would actually suit anyone who has "yo-yo'd" in the past, as this behaviour shows that you do have the self-discipline to stick to a regime for a period of time, and with the Two-Day 5:2 Diet, you only ever have to keep to the regime for a maximum of 24 hours at a time, and you're asleep for about $1/3^{rd}$ of that time!

HOW DOES THE TWO-DAY 5:2 DIET PLAN LEAD TO WEIGHT LOSS?

The 5:2 diet plan **works as your weekly calorie intake is in deficit** compared to what your body needs to maintain your current weight when you combine:

- eating normally but healthily for 5 days
- plus 2 days of restricted calorie intake.

This weekly calorie deficit leads to weight-loss, as long as you **don't treat it as a license to binge on the non-diet days**. What's more, once you have lost weight, you can really **easily maintain that loss** by moving onto a 6:1 regime, meaning that instead of dieting for 2 days a week, you reduce this to just 1 day a week.

Technically, your fast-diet-day calorie allowance should be a quarter of your recommended daily calorie intake. This does vary dependent upon your current weight and level of activity. However, part of the joy of the 5:2 diet plan is its simplicity, and there is a short-cut for this calculation. Most people following the 5:2 diet adopt the plan of sticking to a diet-day allowance of:

- 500 calories for women
- 600 calories for men.

A scientific study published in 2010 (Int J Obes (Lond)) found the Two-Day 5:2 Diet to be as effective at losing weight and improving insulin sensitivity as following a daily calorie-controlled diet. You can reasonably expect that the weekly calorie deficit created by following the Tow-Day 5:2 diet as described above to lead to a **weight loss of 1-2lbs per week**.

Is the Two-Day 5:2 Diet Plan Healthy and is it Suitable for Everyone?

There have been a number of scientific studies that have reported that there are wider health benefits to be gained from a healthy eating plan that incorporates intermittent fasting. Studies have found a correlation between intermittent fasting and lowered blood pressure, lowered cholesterol levels and improvements in insulin sensitivity (Nutrition & Metabolism 2012, Proceedings of the Nutrition Society 2012).

That said you should consult your doctor before commencing a new diet or exercise regime and that includes this plan. In particular, fasting is not suitable for everyone so the 5:2 diet plan **is not suitable for** some people, and particularly it is not appropriate for:

- anyone who is pregnant, planning a pregnancy or breast-feeding
- anyone with a major health condition such as diabetes, irritable bowel syndrome
- anyone who has had an eating disorder.

The Two-Day 5:2 Diet Plan
Diet for Two Days, Feast for Five!
The Easy Three Steps to the Two-Day 5:2 Diet Plan

The plan is so straightforward that it can be explained in just three simple steps, here's what you need to do:

1 At the start of the week, decide which two days are going to be your diet days in that week. A "diet day" is 24 hours long and can start at any point in the day to suit your schedule. You don't need to stick to the same days every week.

2 On your diet day, you must only eat 500 calories (for women) or 600 calories (for men). This needs to cover _everything you eat and drink_ in that 24 hour period.

3 On the other five days, _dine normally and mainly healthily_ (but treats are allowed)! Just remember that the two diet days are there to create a weekly calorie shortfall which leads to weight-loss, so just make sure you **don't overeat on the non-diet days**.

What is the "16 Hour Rule" on the Two-Day 5:2 Diet Plan?

The simple premise of the 5:2 diet is that, twice a week, you just eat 500 or 600 calories within a 24 hr period. Perhaps you have also heard about a "16 hour rule" and wondered what this is? The "16 hour rule" refers to the period of time between the last food eaten on your non-dieting day to the first food eaten on your diet day. Some of the research on the health benefits that can be gained from following a fasting diet regime found that there was a link from extending the period of time of fasting (ie no food consumption at all), especially to a period of 16 hours.

What does this mean in reality? Let's assume that on the day before you diet, you finished eating your evening meal at 7pm and that is the last food you eat that day. Following the "16 hour rule" in this example would mean that you wouldn't eat again on your fast day until 11am ie 16 hrs after 7pm.

Not everyone on the Two-Day 5:2 Diet follows the "16 hour rule", it is unlikely to make much (if any) difference to weight-loss, but it is associated with the wider health benefits related to following an intermittent diet regime.

BREAKFAST, LUNCH AND DINNER?

When you are on your fast-diet-day with calories restricted to 500/600 cals, you need to decide which meals you want to eat. For example, are you going to spread your calorie allowance over the 3 traditional meals of breakfast, lunch and dinner or will you skip a meal and therefore have more calories to spend on the remaining 2 meals?

If you decide to also follow the "16-hour rule", it probably makes sense to skip breakfast altogether and just have lunch and dinner.

However I know many people who feel that they **need to have breakfast** or they just don't have the energy to face the day. Ultimately, how many meals you eat on your fast-diet-days is a matter of personal choice for you, and there is no reason why you can't mix it up, eating 3 meals on some days and 2 on others. This book includes some suggested menu plans for both 500 and 600 calorie days with or without breakfast.

It is also important to carefully count calories on your fast-diet-days. If you just "guestimate" it is all to easy to blow your daily calories allowance, and sticking to 500/600 calories on your fast diet days is key to success on this programme.

Fortunately, this is where **this cookbook comes into play** –an array of tasty, filling, delicious but calorie-counted breakfasts, lunches and dinners –all designed to help you stick to your calorie plan on your diet days.

EATING WELL ON YOUR 5 NON-DIET DAYS

As stated previously, the 5:2 diet is not a license to binge or overeat on your 5 non-diet days. On these days, you will eat normally but healthily. However, what does this actually mean? A healthy balanced diet means eating meals rich in fruit, vegetables, wholegrain cereals and one that is low in saturated fat and salt. However, this doesn't mean foods lacking in taste, flavour or interest –quite the opposite! So, on your non-diet days try to follow this general approach:

eat more:
- fruit and vegetables
- wholegrain breads and cereals,
- pulses (peas, beans and lentils)
- nuts and seeds
- fish, both white and oily varieties

and less:
- high saturated fat dairy
- red meat

To keep the calorie levels very low on the 2 fast-diet days, the recipes for these days are generally very, very low in both total and saturated fat, as fat is very calorie-dense (1g = 9 calories or 1 teaspoon = 45 calories). Whilst it is essential for good health to not regularly eat a lot of saturated fat, it is important to include "good" fats in your diet ie unsaturated fats. These can be found in oily fish, avocado and oils sourced from corn, rapeseed, olives, sunflower seeds and other vegetable, nut and seed oils. They are also present in the vegetable spreads made from those oils. Try to make sure you include some of these great tasting foods in your meals on your non-diet days.

If you are looking for inspiration on cooking normally but healthily on your non-diet days, then you may be interested in my cookbook -**Mediterranean Diet Recipe Cookbook 100+ Heart Healthy Recipes**, this is available on Amazon in both book and Kindle format.

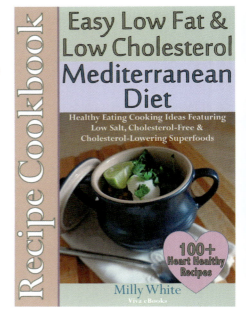

How to Use this Recipe Cookbook

Metric vs American Measurements

All recipes are provided in both Metric and American measurements. In order to provide meaningful equivalents, there may be slight "rounding" differences between the two systems, but these do not make a material difference to the overall calorie count. Egg sizes differ between Europe and the US. All recipes in this book are based on European Medium Eggs which is equivalent to American Large Eggs. Please do not mix Metric and American measurements, especially for baking recipes.

Both European English and American English names have been given for ingredients where they differ in common usage, for example, fresh coriander or fresh cilantro.

Standard **level** spoon measurements are used in all recipes

- 1 tsp = 5ml
- 1 tbsp = 15ml
- A pinch = $^1/_8$ tsp

Individual Ingredient Calorie Counts

The calorie count for individual ingredients has been included in every recipe, which allows the reader to easily adapt the recipe if they do not like or cannot source a specific ingredient. This has been calculated on the metric weight. Additionally, when allocating calories to individual ingredients often there is a need to round up or down, each recipe adds up to its correct recipe total, but there may be slight rounding differences on the calories of an individual ingredient. Again, this does not make a material difference to the overall calorie count.

Vegetarian Recipes & Vegetarian Options

Recipes suitable for vegetarians are indicated with the (V) symbol. In addition, wherever possible in non-vegetarian recipes, alternative vegetarian options have been given on how to adapt the recipe to make it suitable for vegetarians. Where a recipe includes cheese but is indicated with a (V) symbol, it assumes that the cook will use vegetarian cheese if that is required.

Helpful Tips and Tricks for the Two-Day 5:2 Diet Plan

5 Top Tips For Stress-Free Diet Days

1. **Plan ahead** –work out in advance what you are going to eat on your fast days, and buy the ingredients ahead of time. It's not a good plan to be wandering the oh-so-tempting aisles of the supermarket on your fast day, nor to get home after a hard day in the office and be faced with "what should I cook tonight".

2. **Track what you eat** –on the days that you are dieting, make sure you tot-up all your calories and make a note of them. Write them down or track them on your mobile phone or tablet. As well as there not being much of a margin for error on fast days, tracking leads to conscious consumption.

3. **Measure and/or weigh what you eat**. Again, on dieting days, ingredient quantities and portion size are critical; please don't leave it to chance. Take a look at my recommendations for a few simple pieces of equipment that will help enormously in your Diet-Days kitchen.

4. **Keep hydrated**. It's an old adage that often we mistake thirst for hunger. Additionally, proper hydration can help you feel fuller. You can drink water, tea, herb tea, coffee and calorie-free sodas or squashes. Aim to drink 8 good glasses per day (and not just on Fast Days).

5. **Keep occupied**. Make sure you have activities, errands and/or chores planned to occupy your mind on Diet Days. Boredom is also often mistaken for hunger, so keep your mind and fingers busy!

7 Really Useful Diet Day Bits of Kitchen Kit

As previously stated, ingredient quantities and portion control are essential to the low calories of the recipes in this cookbook. Nowadays, we've become so accustomed to large servings, with much more food in a portion than we actually need to be satisfied. However, because the recipes I've developed for this Two-Day 5:2 Diet Plan Cookbook are packed full of natural, flavoursome ingredients, the recommended portion-sizes will leaving you feeling full and satisfied, even on your dieting days.

The following pieces of kitchen-ware can really help with keeping portion sizes under control.

1. A standard set of measuring spoons: 1/8th tsp to 1 tbsp
2. A standard set of cup measures: ¼ cup, 1/3 cup, 1/2 cup, 1 cup
3. A set of digital kitchen scales
4. A small measuring jug
5. Chopping board
6. Vegetable peeler
7. Mini food processor

THE TWO-DAY 5:2 DIET PLAN PANTRY

Often we associate low-calorie, low-fat food with being tasteless and unsatisfying, and you still feel hungry and wanting more after you've eaten it . I think this is especially true when eating shop-bought *diet foods* as they are often packed full of artificial ingredients and flavourings. That is not the case with the recipes in this book, which are brimming with natural ingredients that boost the flavour-factor but not the calorie-count. To do this, it's helpful to have your pantry well-stocked with these ingredients. You don't need to buy them all in one go, but try to build them up over time.

- a variety of dried herbs and spices: oregano, basil, mint, rosemary, parsley, cumin, ground coriander, cinnamon
- a variety of dried and canned beans and lentils
- hot pepper sauce such as Tabasco
- tinned tomatoes
- soy sauce
- sea salt or kosher salt
- fresh ground pepper
- cornflour (corn starch)
- Frylight olive oil spray
- capers
- gherkins
- sauerkraut
- Swiss vegetable bouillon powder
- reduced salt stock cubes
- mustard (powder & Dijon)

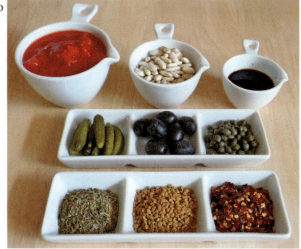

I also have a little indoor kitchen herb garden that includes my most often used fresh herbs - thyme, basil, mint, parsley and coriander, and I just harvest the leaves I need to complete my dish.

Example Day Menu Planners
500 calorie Example Menu Plans

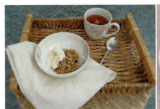 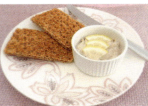 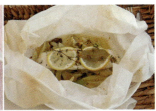

Menus with Breakfast, Lunch & Dinner

Example 1: Total Calories In Menu = 484
  Breakfast: *5:2 Nutty Maple Granola*
  Lunch: *Smoked Mackerel Pâté & Crisp Breads*
  Dinner: *Garlic & Herb Roasted Cod with Fennel En Papillote*

Example 2: Total Calories In Menu = 498
  Breakfast: *Creamy Peppered Mushrooms on Toast*
  Lunch: *Red Pepper & Roasted Garlic Humous with Crudités*
  Dinner: *Tuna Niçoise Salad*

Example 3: Total Calories In Menu = 477
  Breakfast: *New Yorker Deli Breakfast Slice*
  Lunch: *Superfood Soup*
  Dinner: *Turkey Pot Pie*

Menus with Lunch & Dinner

Example 1: Total Calories In Menu = 500
  Lunch: *Grilled Ruben Sandwich*
  Dinner: *Tandoori Chicken Kebabs with Brown Basmati Rice*

Example 2: Total Calories In Menu = 421
  Lunch: *Red Pepper & Cottage Cheese Frittata*
  Dinner: *Mushroom Stroganoff with Basmati Rice*

Example 3: Total Calories In Menu = 464
  Lunch: *Spicy Roasted Vegetables and Humous Pitta*
  Dinner: *Aromatic Duck with Plum Sauce & Sautéed Cabbage with Basmati Rice*

600 CALORIE EXAMPLE MENU PLANS

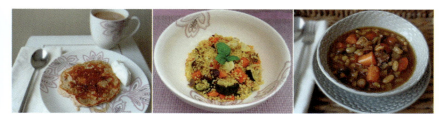

MENUS WITH BREAKFAST, LUNCH & DINNER

Example 1: Total Calories In Menu = 595
  Breakfast: Cinnamon Apple Pie Pancakes
  Lunch: Mediterranean Cous Cous Salad
  Dinner: Ragout of Lamb and Beans

Example 2: Total Calories In Menu = 589
  Breakfast: "Full English Breakfast" Frittata
  Lunch: Red Pepper & Roasted Garlic Humous with Crudités
  Dinner: Choucroute Garni with Mustard Cream Sauce

Example 3: Total Calories In Menu = 619
  Breakfast: Peach Parfait Smoothie
  Lunch: Tuna 'Mayo' Sandwich
  Dinner: Parma-Wrapped Chicken & Garlicky Roast Potatoes

MENUS WITH LUNCH & DINNER

Example 1: Total Calories In Menu = 532
  Lunch: Grilled Ruben Sandwich
  Dinner: Individual Cottage Pies with steamed new potatoes

Example 2: Total Calories In Menu = 545
  Lunch: Smoked Mackerel Pâté & Crisp Breads
  Dinner: Choucroute Garni with Mustard Cream Sauce with steamed new potatoes

Example 3: Total Calories In Menu = 536
  Lunch: Tuna 'Mayo' Sandwich
  Dinner: Turkey Pot Pie with steamed new potatoes

Two-Day 5:2 Diet Breakfasts

Two-Day 5:2 Diet Breakfasts
100 Calories & Under

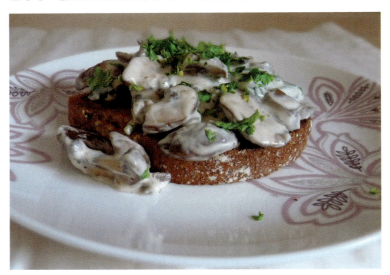

Creamy Peppered Mushrooms on Toast (V)

Ingredients with cals per serving

- 120g (1 cup) chestnut (baby portabella) mushrooms –10 cals
- 35g (2 tbsp + 1 tsp) 3% fat soft cheese –20 cals
- ½ tsp freshly ground black pepper
- ½ tsp flat leaf parsley, chopped 1 cal
- 2 sprays Frylight olive oil spray- 2 cal
- 2 small slices calorie controlled brown bread eg Weight Watchers –48 cal

Directions

Clean the mushrooms then slice. Heat a large skillet over a medium heat and spritz with two sprays of Frylight olive oil spray. Add the mushrooms and cook until browned. Meanwhile toast the bread. Remove mushrooms from heat and stir in the soft cheese and freshly ground black pepper. Stir until soft cheese has fully melted, then divide the Creamy Peppered Mushrooms mixture over the toast slices and sprinkle with chopped flat leaf parsley.

Serves: 2   Ready In: 5 mins   Per Serving: 83 Calories

New Yorker Deli Breakfast Slice

Ingredients with cals per serving

- 2 Ryvita rye crackers - 35 cals
- 60g (¼ cup) low fat cottage cheese - 19 cals
- 30g (2) small slices smoked salmon - 30 cals
- 3 cocktail gherkins - 3 cals
- ½ tsp baby capers, drained - 1 cals
- ¼ whole English cucumber - 4 cals
- 1 medium tomato - 5 cals
- pinch freshly ground pepper

Directions

Rinse the capers and pat dry. Finely chop them along with the cocktail gherkins and mix into the cottage cheese, along with a good grinding of fresh black pepper. Thinly slice the cucumber. Halve the tomato, scoop out the seeds and discard, and then chop the tomato flesh into small dice. Cut the smoked salmon into thin strips.

Assemble by dividing the cottage cheese mixture over the two rye crackers. Top first with the smoked salmon slices, then the cucumber, and finally the diced tomato. Finish a twist of ground pepper.

Serves: 2   Ready In: 5 mins   Per Serving: 97 Calories

SuperBlue Smoothie (V)

Ingredients with cals per serving

- 120mls (½ cup) fresh skimmed (low fat) milk –21 cals
- 120g (½ cup) low fat soya yogurt - 30 cals
- 75g (½ cup) blueberries, fresh or frozen   - 20 cals
- 1 tsp honey –10 cals
- 2 tsp wheatgerm –19 cals

Directions

Place all the ingredients into a blender and whizz together until smooth. Pour into 2 glasses and serve.

Serves: 2   Ready In: 2 mins   Per Serving: 100 Calories

Hashed Brown Potato Cake With Mushroom & Tomato (V)

Ingredients with cals per serving

- 2 medium red potatoes (200g) –78 cals
- 2 flat mushrooms (63g) –5 cals
- ½ beef tomato (90g), cut into 2 thick slices –9 cals
- 2 medium spring onions/scallions (40g) –5 cals
- 2 sprays Frylight olive oil spray - 1 cal
- 1 tsp fresh thyme, chopped –1 cal
- pinch sea (kosher) salt
- pinch freshly ground black pepper

Directions

Grate the potatoes (skin on) onto a clean tea towel or kitchen towel, and then squeeze really hard to remove the juice. Pat dry with fresh kitchen towel and place in a bowl. Remove the leaves from the fresh thyme (discard the woody stalks) and shred finely, along with the spring onions. Reserve a pinch of thyme/onion for serving, then add the remaining to the potatoes. Season with salt and black pepper and mix well. Divide the mixture into two, and squeeze each portion between the palms of your hands to form a patty shape.

Preheat a non-stick sauté pan. Spritz with a spray of Frylight olive oil spray and add the potato cakes to the hot pan. After 5 minutes, turn the cakes over. Spritz the pan again with another spray of Frylight olive oil spray and add the mushrooms. After 3 minutes, turn the mushrooms and add the tomato slices. Cook for a further 2 minutes. Serve each Hashed Brown Potato Cake topped with a slice of tomato and a mushroom. Sprinkle with the reserved thyme/onion.

Serves: 2   Ready In: 10 mins   Per Serving: 99 Calories

Two-Day 5:2 Diet Breakfasts 150 Calories & Under

5:2 Nutty Maple Granola (V)

Ingredients with cals per serving

- ½ tsp olive oil –2 cals
- 1 tbsp pure maple syrup –4 cals
- 40ml (3 tbsp) apple juice (apple cider) –2 cals
- 90g (1 cup) quick cook rolled oats –34 cals
- 20g (¼ cup) wheat flakes –8 cals
- 25g (¼ cup) barley flakes –9 cals
- 15g (1 tbsp) rye flakes –5 cals
- 15g (1 tbsp) pumpkin seeds –9 cals
- 15g (1 tbsp) sweetened desiccated coconut –9 cals
- 6 dried apricot halves (20g) –4 cals
- 2 tsp currants (10g) –3 cals
- 10 pecan nut halves (15g) –10 cals
- 15g (1 ½ tbsp) flaked almonds –9 cals
- 50mls (1/5 cup) 0% fat Greek yogurt (per serving) –28 cals

Directions

Preheat the oven to 140C fan, 300F, Gas Mark 4. Line a baking sheet with parchment.

Chop the apricot halves and pecan nuts. In a large bowl, mix together all the dry ingredients. Mix the oil, maple syrup and apple juice in a jug and pour over the dry mix. Stir well to ensure that all the ingredients are wet. Spread onto a baking sheet and place into the oven. Bake for a total of 45-60 mins, checking every 15 mins and turning it over. The granola is ready when it is all toasted and dry.

Remove from oven and allow to cool completely. Store in a sealed container. Makes 10 servings and will keep for 3 months in a sealed container.

Serve 1 portion with 50mls ($1/5$ cup) of 0% Fat Greek yogurt.

Serves: 10 **Ready In:** 1hr 15 mins **Per Serving:** 136 Calories

Peach Parfait Smoothie (V)

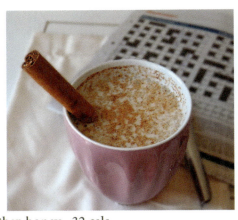

Ingredients with cals per serving
- 120mls (½ cup) fresh skimmed (low fat) milk –21 cals
- 120g (½ cup) 0% fat Greek yogurt –34 cals
- 120g (½ cup) sliced peaches in juice, drained –25 cals
- ½ medium banana (75g) –17 cals
- ¼ tsp vanilla bean paste –2 cals
- pinch freshly grated nutmeg
- 1 tbsp honey –32 cals
- 2 tsp wheatgerm –19 cals

Directions
Place all the ingredients except the nutmeg into a blender and whizz together until smooth. Pour into 2 glasses & grate over the nutmeg.

Serves: 2   Ready In: 2 mins   Per Serving: 150 Calories

Banana & Walnut TeaBread (V)

Ingredients with cals per serving
- 175g (1½ cup) wholemeal (whole-wheat) flour –48 cals
- 20g (3 tbsp) walnut halves, chopped – 11 cals
- 75g (⅓ cup) light brown sugar, packed –24 cals
- 2 UK med (US large) free range eggs– 15 cals
- 2 tsp baking powder
- ¼ tsp bicarbonate of soda (baking soda)
- 75g (½ stick + 1 tbsp) lighter spreadable (reduced fat) butter –34 cals
- 1 tbsp honey –5 cals
- 1½ medium ripe bananas (225g) –13 cals

Directions
Preheat the oven to 160C fan, 350F, Gas Mark 6. Line a 450g/1lb loaf tin with baking parchment. Mix together the flour, baking and bicarbonate of soda (baking soda) and set to one side. With an electric food mixer, beat together the butter, sugar and honey until light and fluffy. Beat in the eggs, one at a time. Mix in the mashed bananas. With the food mixer on low, gently add the flour and chopped walnut halves, taking care not to over beat the mixture at this stage.Spoon into the tin and bake for about 1 hour or until a wooden skewer comes out clean. Leave to cool in the tin for 15 mins then turn out to finish cooling on a rack. When cold, slice into 12 slices.

Prepare & Freeze Tip: Wrap individual slices in greaseproof (waxed) paper and place in freezer bags to store. Defrost individual slices overnight for breakfast.

Serves: 12   Ready In: 90 mins   Per Serving: 150 Calories

Breakfast Bars (V)

Ingredients with cals per serving

- 70g (½ cup) toasted wheat germ –13 cals
- 30g (¼ cup) wholemeal (whole-wheat) flour –5 cals
- 90g (1 cup) quick cook rolled oats -18 cals
- 35g (½ cup) powdered non-fat dry milk –6 cals
- 45g (1/3 cup) pumpkin seeds –14 cals
- 75g (½ cup) dried ready to eat apricots –10 cals
- 65g (½ cup) pecan nut halves –24 cals
- 200g (½ cup) dried cranberries –13 cals
- 100g (½ cup) pitted dried dates, whole –15 cals
- 1 medium ripe banana (150g) –7 cals
- 2 UK med (US large) free range eggs –9 cals
- 1 tsp vanilla bean paste –1 cal
- ½ tsp ground cinnamon
- 60mls (¼ cup) pure maple syrup - 12

Directions

Preheat the oven to 180C fan, 375F, Gas Mark 6. Line a 23cm x 33cm (9x13in) baking tin with baking parchment.

Roughly chop the pecan nuts, dried apricots, dates and cranberries (you can pulse this in a food processor to save time, but it will result in a less "chunky" bar). In a large bowl, mash the banana with a fork. Mix in the eggs, one at a time. Stir in the maple syrup, ground cinnamon and vanilla bean paste. Add the chopped fruits and nuts and the pumpkin seeds. Stir well. Finally, fold in the cooled toasted wheatgerm, flour, oats and dried milk powder.

Press the mixture into the lined baking tin, and bake in the pre-heated oven for 20 mins. Remove from the oven and leave to cool in the tin. When completely cooled, remove from tin and cut into 20 even sized pieces.

Prepare & Freeze Tip: Wrap individual bars in greaseproof (waxed) paper and place in freezer bags to store. Defrost a bar overnight for breakfast the following day.

Serves: 20   Ready In: 35 mins   Per Serving: 147 Calories

Two-Day 5:2 Diet Breakfasts 200 Calories & Under

Cheesy Baked Eggs Florentine (V)

Ingredients with cals per serving
- 250g (8 cups) raw spinach –30 cals
- ½ tbsp cornflour/corn starch –13 cals
- ½ tsp dry mustard powder –4 cals
- ½ tsp Swiss vegetable bouillon powder –4 cals
- 2 UK med (US large) free range eggs –88 cals
- 1½ tbsp (10g) grated low fat mature cheese –14 cals
- 100ml (½ cup) semi skimmed (1.8% fat) fresh milk –25 cal
- pinch ground black pepper , sea (kosher) salt and freshly ground nutmeg

Directions
Preheat the oven to 180C fan, 375F, Gas Mark 6. Rinse the spinach in a colander and shake off excess moistures. Heat a non-stick saucepan over a medium heat and add the spinach. Season with freshly ground black pepper and a pinch of salt. Cook until wilted. Use a slotted spoon and divide evenly between two oven-proof ramekins, creating a well in the centre of each portion. Rinse the pan out. Mix the cornflour (corn starch) with a little of the milk to a smooth paste. Heat the remaining milk in the saucepan over a medium heat. Stir in the paste; whisking until the sauce thickens. Add the stock powder, mustard powder and nutmeg. Crack one egg into each of the wells in the spinach. Spoon over the sauce and sprinkle with the grated cheese. Bake in a preheated oven for 10-12 mins, until the eggs are cooked to you liking.

Serves: 2   Ready In: 20 mins   Per Serving: 179 Calories

Bircher Muesli (V)

Ingredients with cals per serving
- 45g (½ cup) quick cook rolled oats –86 cals
- 100ml (½ cup) plain fat-free yogurt –31 cals
- 2 tsp pure maple syrup or honey –18 cals
- 2 tsp fresh lemon juice –2 cals
- 1 medium apple (135g) –40 cals
- 1 ½ tbsp (15g) seedless raisins -22 cals

Directions
Mix together the oats, raisins, yogurt and maple syrup/honey. Seal and leave in the fridge overnight. In the morning, grate the apple (skin on) and toss in lemon juice. Fold into the oat mixture, divide into two bowls and serve.

Serves: 2   Ready In: 5 mins   Per Serving: 199 Calories

Full English Breakfast Frittata

Ingredients with cals per serving

- 7 cherry tomatoes (80g) –8 cals
- 2 smoked turkey rashers –27 cals
- 3 small new potatoes (127g/4 ½ oz) –48 cals
- 60g (½ cup) chestnut (baby portabella) mushrooms –8 cals
- 2 UK med (US large) free range eggs - 88 cals
- 2 UK med (US large) free range egg whites - 17 cals
- 3 sprays Frylight olive oil spray –1 cal
- ½ tsp flat leaf parsley, chopped
- pinch ground black pepper and sea (kosher) salt

Directions

Wash the potatoes then chop into dice (skins still on). Microwave in a container with 2 tbsp of water and a very small pinch of salt for 2 mins then drain. Heat a heavy-bottom non-stick sauté pan to medium high. Spritz with 2 sprays of Frylight spray and add the potato. Cook for 2-3 mins until starting to brown.

Slice the rashers into strips and add to the pan. Meanwhile, wipe the mushrooms clean and slice. Add to the non-stick sauté pan and continue to cook, turning the ingredients to prevent burning, until the mushrooms are golden. Halve the tomatoes.

Preheat the grill to medium.

In a bowl, whisk together the 2 whole eggs and 2 egg whites until frothy. Season with freshly ground black pepper and salt. Spray the non-stick sauté pan with one more spritz of Frylight oil. Add the egg mixture, tipping the pan so that it covers the base. Turn down the heat and scatter over the tomato halves. Cook for 6 minutes, or until almost set. Place under the preheated grill, for 2-3 minutes, until the frittata is set and golden. Let cool slightly, then slide out of the pan, cut into wedges, sprinkle with chopped parsley and serve.

Vegetarian Option: Substitute the smoked turkey rashers with Quorn bacon-style slices instead. Calories per serving 190

Serves: 2   Ready In: 20 mins   Per Serving: 197 Calories

Cinnamon Apple Pie Pancakes (V)

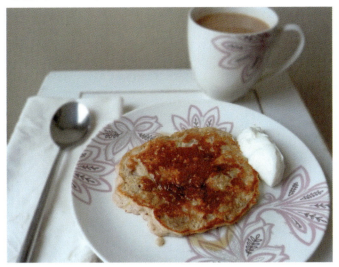

Ingredients with cals per serving

- 100g (¹/₃ cup + 1 tbsp) low fat buttermilk –20 cals
- 45g (¹/₃ cup) wholemeal (whole-wheat) flour –77 cals
- 1 tsp natural caster sugar –9 cals
- ½ tsp baking powder
- ¼ tsp bicarbonate of soda (baking soda)
- ½ tsp ground cinnamon –1 cal
- 1 UK med (US large) free range egg, separated –44 cals
- 1 small eating apple, grated (85g) –23 cals
- 1 tbsp seedless raisins –13 cals
- 4 sprays 1-cal butter spray –2 cals
- 2 tbsp 0% fat Greek yogurt –9 cals

Directions

Sieve together the flour, baking powder and baking soda into a bowl. Mix in the caster sugar. In a separate clean bowl, whisk the egg white until stiff.

Combine the egg yolk with the buttermilk in a jug, and then pour into the flour/sugar mixture. With a fork, whisk until smooth. Grate the apple (skin on) and add to the mixture along with the raisins. Finally, carefully fold in the stiff egg white.

Heat a large frying pan and spray with 2 spritz of the 1-cal Butter Spray. Drop in spoonfuls of batter, so each pancake is about ¼ of the mixture. Cook for 2 minutes each side until cooked through. Remove and keep warm. Repeat to make 4 pancakes.

Serve 2 pancakes with 1 tbsp of 0% Greek yogurt.

Serves: 2   Ready In: 15 mins   Per Serving: 198 Calories

Two-day 5:2 Diet Lunches

150 Calories & Under

Stuffed Peppers Provençale

Ingredients with cals per serving

- 2 red bell peppers –50 cals
- 4 cherry tomatoes (45g) –6 cals
- 4 artichoke hearts (tinned or frozen, not oil, 88g) –11 cals
- 4 black olives, drained (10g) - 8 cals
- 2 anchovy fillets, rinsed and drained (8g) –8 cals
- 2 tbsp fresh basil, cut into strips –1 cal
- 2 sprays Frylight olive oil spray –1 cal
- pinch ground black pepper and sea (kosher) salt

Directions

Preheat the oven to 180C fan, 375F, Gas Mark 6.

Start by rinsing well all the canned foods (artichoke hearts, olives, anchovy fillets) to remove canning brine and salt, and then pat dry on kitchen towel.

With a sharp kitchen knife, cut each pepper in half through the stalk. Remove the pith and seeds and discard but keep the stalk in place as it will help keep the peppers in shape when cooking. Transfer the halves, cut sides up, into a roasting tin.

Cut in half the artichoke hearts, olives and tomatoes and distribute evenly between the 4 pepper halves. Chop up the anchovy fillets and pop them into gaps in the stuffed peppers. Finally, chiffonade (cut into thin strips) the basil leaves, scatter over the stuffed peppers and spritz them with 2 sprays of Frylight olive oil spray.

Cover the roasting tin loosely with tin foil and bake in the oven for 25 mins.

The peppers can be served immediately hot from the oven, or allowed to cool and served at room temperature for a packed lunch.

Vegetarian Option: Omit the anchovy fillets. Calories per serving 75.

Serves: 2   **Ready In:** 30 mins   **Per Serving:** 83 Calories

CRUNCHY SESAME DUCK & ORANGE SALAD

Ingredients with cals per serving

- 125g (4 ½ oz) skinless duck breast fillet –58 cals
- ½ English cucumber (90g) –5 cals
- 2 large spring onions/scallions (40g) –5 cals
- 100g (1 cup) beansprouts (mung) –17 cals
- 1 tsp toasted sesame seeds –9 cals
- 100g (1 cup) Chinese leaf/Nappa cabbage, chopped –7 cals
- ½ tbsp rice wine vinegar - 1 cal
- 1 tsp fresh lime juice –1 cal
- ½ tsp toasted sesame oil –10 cals
- 1 easy peeler Clementine –18 cals
- 2 sprays Frylight spray –1 cal
- pinch black pepper and sea salt
- 1 tbsp Hoisin sauce –13 cals

Directions

If you using raw sesame seeds, then start by toasting them in a non-stick sauté pan over a medium heat. Keep tossing the seeds, watching closely and remove from pan as soon as they are toasted. Cut the duck breast into strips, then season with salt and black pepper. Preheat a non-stick sauté pan and cook in the pan for 5 mins on each side. Remove the pan from the heat and allow the duck to rest for few mins. Meanwhile, chop the cucumber and spring onion (scallion) and mix in a large bowl together with the salad leaf and beansprouts. Divide between two dinner plates. Peel the Clementine, segment and scatter over the salad. In a small jug, whisk together the Hoisin sauce, rice wine vinegar, lime juice and toasted sesame oil. Pour over the duck strips (still in the pan) and toss together. Spoon the duck and dressing over the salad and serve.

Vegetarian Option: Replace the duck with chicken-style Quorn, cals per serving 141

Serves: 2   Ready In: 15 mins   Per Serving: 143 Calories

CHICKEN VERONIQUE LETTUCE CUPS

Ingredients with cals per serving

- 100g (3½ oz) roasted chicken breast –53 cals
- 1 tbsp lighter than light mayonnaise –5 cals
- 1 tbsp 0% Greek yogurt –4 cals
- 50g (¹/₃ cup) seedless green grapes –18 cals
- ½ tbsp fresh tarragon, chopped
- 50g (½ cup) fennel bulb –5 cals
- ½ baby gem lettuce head –4 cals
- pinch black pepper and sea salt

Directions

Shred the skinless roasted chicken and halve the grapes. Slice the fennel really thinly. In a bowl, mix together the mayonnaise, yogurt and tarragon (use ½ tsp of dried if you don't have fresh) and season to taste with salt and pepper. Add the shredded chicken, grapes and fennel, and stir well to coat everything in the dressing. Separate the leaves of the gem lettuce. Rinse and dry. Spoon the chicken mixture into the lettuce leaves.

Vegetarian Option: Replace the chicken with chicken-style Quorn, cals per serving 96.

Serves: 2   Ready In: 5 mins   Per Serving: 89 Calories

SUPERFOOD SOUP (V)

Ingredients with cals per serving

- 150g (1 ½ cup) fennel bulb, chopped –3 cals
- 300g (10oz) frozen garden peas –26 cals
- 200g ($1^{1}/_{3}$) cup frozen podded soya edamame beans –32 cals
- 250g (8 cups) raw spinach –7 cals
- 100g (1 cup) leek, sliced –3 cals
- 3 vegetable stock cubes –12 cals
- 2 tbsp mint leaves, chopped –1 cal
- 1 medium garlic bulb –5 cals
- pinch ground black pepper and sea (kosher) salt

Directions

Preheat the oven to 180C fan, 375F, Gas Mark 6. Using a sharp knife, slice the top off the garlic bulb, then wrap in a piece of kitchen foil and place directly onto the oven rack in the centre and cook for 20 minutes. (Tip - This can be done in advance when you have the oven on for something else and will store (wrapped) in the fridge for up to 4 days before use). Allow to cool enough to handle.

Meanwhile, in a large saucepan, dissolve the 3 stock cubes in 1 litre (1 quart) of boiling water. Reserve 50gs ($^{1}/_{3}$ cup) of peas and beans mixed, and put to one side. Chop the fennel and leek and add to the stock along with the peas and edamame beans. Bring back to the boil and simmer gently for 10 minutes. Add the raw spinach, return to simmer for a further 5 mins. Unwrap the baked garlic and squeeze out the roasted garlic paste into the soup, along with the chopped mint (I wear clean rubber kitchen gloves when I do this as it can be messy!). Allow soup to cool slightly then pour into a food processor and whizz to a smooth consistency. You may well need to do this in 2-3 batches dependent on the capacity of your food processor, or alternatively use a stick processor to blend directly in the pan. Return to the blended soup to the pan, add back the reserved peas/beans and season to taste. Re-warm to serve.

A serving is 250g/1 cup. Freeze individual portions to keep, then defrost and microwave on high for 3½ mins to serve.

Serves: 8   **Ready In:** 25 mins   **Per Serving:** 89 Calories

Red Pepper & Roasted Garlic Humous with Crudités (V)

Ingredients with cals per serving
- 1 red bell pepper −8 cals
- 1 small garlic bulb −4 cals
- 2 tsp tahini paste −10 cals
- 100g (½ cup) 0% Greek yogurt −10 cals
- 1 lemon, squeezed −2 cals
- 240g (1½ cups) tinned, drained chickpeas - 48 cals
- pinch ground black pepper

per serving to accompany
- 1 Italian breadstick −21 cals
- ½ celery stick −3 cals
- 1 medium carrot −25 cals

Directions

Preheat the oven to 180C fan, 375F, Gas Mark 6. Using a sharp knife, slice the top off the garlic bulb, then wrap in a piece of kitchen foil and place directly onto a baking sheet along with the red pepper in the centre and cook for 25 mins. Remove from oven. Transfer the red pepper into a heat-proof bowl and cover with cling wrap. Once cool, you will be able to rub/peel off the skin of the red pepper, discard the peel, seeds and stalk, just leaving the pepper flesh.

Rinse the tinned chickpeas well under cold running water, drain fully and then place into a food processor. Add the cooked pepper, tahini paste, Greek yogurt and lemon juice. Unwrap the baked garlic and squeeze out the roasted garlic paste into the processor (I wear clean rubber kitchen gloves when I do this as it can be messy!). Blend until smooth. Season to taste with black pepper and a dash or two of Tabasco if you like a little more kick.

A serving is about 80g or 4 tablespoons. Divide into 6 individual ramekins and chill for 2 hours before serving. To keep, freeze individual portions (use within 3 months). Defrost overnight in the fridge.

Serve a portion with 1 Italian Breadstick, ½ a celery stick and a small carrot (both cut into batons).

Serves: 6   Ready In: 30 mins   Per Serving: 131 Calories

Red Pepper & Cottage Cheese Frittatas (V)

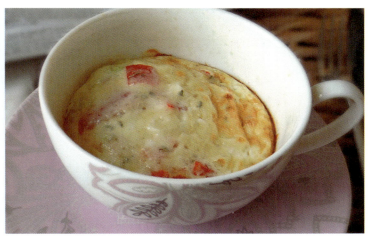

Ingredients
- ½ red bell pepper –13 cals
- 2 UK large (US extra large) free range eggs –103 cals
- 1 UK large (US extra large) free range egg white - 10 cals
- 4 tbsp fat free cottage cheese –22 cals
- 2 scallions (spring onions), sliced –5 cals
- 2 tsp freshly chopped parsley
- 2 sprays Frylight olive oil spray
- pinch freshly grated nutmeg
- pinch kosher/sea salt

Directions
Preheat the oven to 180C fan, 350F, Gas Mark 6. Spray 2 oven-proof ramekins with a spray of olive oil spray. Deseed the red pepper and slice along with the spring onions. Finely chop the parsley. In a jug, break in the whole eggs and add the egg white. Season with kosher/sea salt and a generous grating of nutmeg and lightly whisk. Fold in the cottage cheese, sliced red pepper, spring onions (scallions) and chopped parsley. Divide the mixture between the ramekins. Bake for 18-20 mins or until puffy and just set. These can be eaten hot from the oven, warm or cold (so great for lunch on the go).

Serves: 2   Ready In: 20 mins   Per Serving: 85 Calories

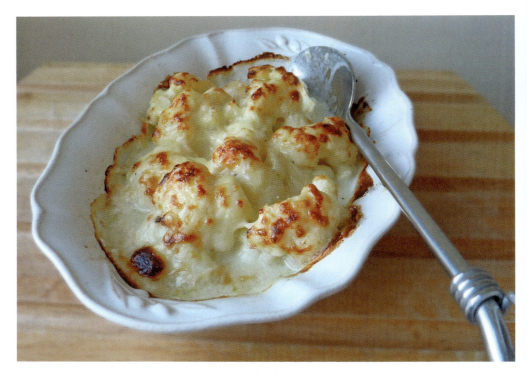

Cauliflower Gratin (V)

Ingredients with cals per serving
- 300g (3 cups) cauliflower florets −57 cals
- 120mls (½ cup) semi-skimmed (reduced fat) milk −35 cals
- 20g (3 tbsp) grated 50% reduced fat mature cheddar cheese −28 cals
- 7g (1 tbsp) finely grated fresh parmesan cheese −9 cals
- ½ tsp dry mustard powder −3 cals
- 1 tbsp cornflour/corn starch −14 cals
- pinch ground black pepper and sea (kosher) salt

Directions
Preheat the oven to 180C fan, 375F, Gas Mark 6.

Lightly steam the cauliflower florets for 5 mins, then transfer to an ovenproof dish.

Meanwhile, in a small bowl, slacken (dissolve) the cornflour (corn starch) with a little of the cold milk. Heat the rest of the milk until just before simmering, stir the dissolved corn starch again to make sure that it is still fully dissolved then quickly whisk the mixture into the hot milk. Continue whisking until the sauce thickens, then allow to simmer gentle for 1 min. Whisk in the mustard powder and the grated cheeses. Stir until cheese has melted and season with salt and pepper to taste.

Pour over the cauliflower florets and bake in the oven until golden brown.

Serves: 2 Ready In: 25 mins   Per Serving: 146 Calories

5:2 Lunches 200 Calories & Under

Smoked Mackerel Pâté & Crisp Breads

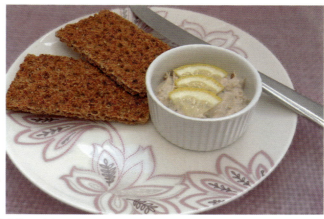

Ingredients with cals per serving
- 250g (9 oz) smoked mackerel fillets (skinned) –73 cals
- 250g (1 cup) 3% fat soft cheese – 29 cals
- 30g (1 tbsp) pickled cocktail cornichons, drained and rinsed – 1 cals
- 10g 2 tsp pickled baby capers, drained and rinsed –1 cals
- ½ lemon, squeezed
- pinch ground black pepper

Per serving to accompany :
- 2 Ryvita cracked pepper crisp breads –76 cals

Directions

Roughly chop the cocktail gherkins and baby capers, and then place into a food processor and pulse. Remove any skin or bones from the smoked mackerel fillets. Add to processor along with the cheese, lemon juice and black pepper. Blend until smooth. A serving is 50g or 3 tbsp. Divide into 10 individual ramekins and chill for 2 hours before serving. To keep, freeze individual portions (use within 3 months). Defrost overnight in the fridge. Serve a portion with 2 Ryvita cracked pepper crisp breads.

Serves: 10 Ready In: 25 mins [Plus chilling time] Per Serving: 180 Calories

Tuna 'Mayo' Sandwich

Ingredients with cals per serving
- 60g (2 oz) no-drain, canned, pole and line-caught tuna (not in oil) –68 cals
- 20g (1 tbsp + 1 tsp) 3% fat soft cheese –23 cals
- 20g (½ cup) fresh watercress –5 cals
- whole-wheat sandwich thin –100 cals

Directions

Flake the tuna fish into a bowl and combine with the cheese. Open the sandwich thin and fill with tuna mix and watercress. Sandwich thin together and serve.

Serves: 1 Ready In: 5 mins Per Serving: 196 Calories

Spicy Roasted Vegetables and Humous Pitta (V)

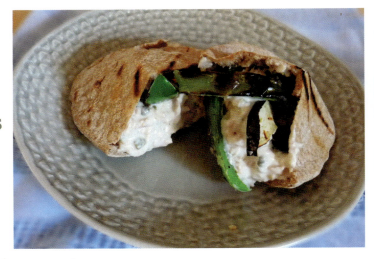

Ingredients with cals per serving

- 2 wholemeal mini pitta –74 cal
- 75g (²/₃ cup) courgette/zucchini –7 cals
- ½ red bell pepper, sliced –13 cals
- 1 salad tomato (80g) –8 cals
- 50g (½ cup fennel) bulb, sliced –9 cals
- ½ small red onion, sliced (35g) –7 cals
- ½ tsp dried mixed herbs
- ½ bag mixed salad leaves –5 cals
- 4 pitted black olives, drained –8 cals
- 1 tsp tomato puree –3 cals
- ½ lemon, squeezed –2 cals
- ½ tsp ground cumin powder –2 cals
- ¼ tsp ground cayenne powder
- 2 dashes Tabasco sauce
- 20g (1 tbsp) reduced fat humous –26 cals
- 1 tsp baby capers, drained –1 cals
- pinch ground black pepper
- pinch sea (kosher) salt
- 1 garlic clove –1 cal
- 4 sprays Frylight olive oil spray –2 cals

Directions

Preheat the oven to 180C fan, 375F, Gas Mark 6 and place a non-stick roasting tin on a high shelf to warm.

Mix together the slices of courgette (zucchini), pepper, fennel and onion. Finely chop the garlic. Spray the vegetables with 4 spritzs of the Frylight spray, sprinkle with chopped garlic, dried herbs, salt and pepper. Spread onto the pre-heated roasting tin in a single layer and return tin to oven. Roast for 25-30 mins. Meanwhile, mix together the tomato puree, lemon juice, Tabasco sauce, cumin and cayenne pepper. Slice the olives and chop the baby capers. When ready, remove the roasted vegetables from the oven. Put the pitta breads into the hot oven for 2 mins to puff up. Toss the warm vegetables with the dressing, olives and capers.

Carefully remove the hot pitta breads from the oven, split open and spread with the reduced fat humous. Divide the salad mix between the pittas and top with the spicy roasted vegetables.

Serves: 2   Ready In: 10 mins   Per Serving: 168 Calories

Grilled Ruben Sandwich

Ingredients with cals per serving
- 28g (1 oz) thinly sliced pastrami −32 cals
- 15g (1 tbsp) 3% fat soft cheese −17 cals
- 2 tbsp sauerkraut, −3 cals
- 10g (1 ½ tbsp) grated 50% reduced fat mature cheddar cheese −28 cals
- 1 tsp tomato ketchup −5 cals
- 1 dill pickle, sliced -12 cals
- 1 soft brown sandwich thin −100 cals

Directions
Preheat the grill or health grill. Rinse and drain the pickle and sauerkraut to remove excess salt. Mix together the ketchup and soft cheese, divide the sandwich thin and spread with the mixture. Onto one of the sandwich thin halves, layer up the sauerkraut, pastrami, dill pickle slices and grated cheese. Top with the remaining sandwich thin half and secure with a cocktail stick. Cook the sandwiches for 2-3 minutes in a health grill or cook for 2 minutes each side under a cooker grill.

Vegetarian Option: Substitute the pastrami with Quorn peppered beef slices instead. Calories per serving 194

Serves: 1   Ready In: 10 mins   Per Serving: 197 Calories

Sweet Chilli Prawn Stir Fry

Ingredients with cals per serving
- 60g (2/3 cup) Chinese leaf /Nappa cabbage, chopped −8 cals
- 60g (½ cup) mange tout (snow peas) −10 cals
- 50g (1/3 cup) frozen edamame beans −31 cals
- 60g (½ cup) beansprouts (mung) −9 cals
- 100g (1 cup) chestnut (baby portabella) mushrooms −8 cals
- 100g (2/3 cup) cooked king prawn/shrimp −40 cals
- 60g (½ cup) baby corn −10 cals
- 1 medium carrot (60g) - 9 cals
- 2 tbsp Thai sweet chilli sauce −28 cals
- 1 garlic clove −1 cal
- ½ red bell pepper −12 cals
- 2 sprays Frylight olive oil spray −1 cal
- pinch sea (kosher) salt

Directions
Cut the carrot and bell pepper into strips. Clean the mushrooms and slice. Halve the mange tout and baby corn. Heat up a wok over a medium heat and spritz twice with Frylight spray. Start stir frying the peppers, mushrooms, carrot and baby corn. After 3 mins, add in the remaining vegetables and continue stir frying for another 3 mins. Add the soya beans and prawns and continue to cook until the beans have fully defrosted and the prawns have warmed through completely. Remove from heat and stir through the Thai sweet chilli sauce. Season with salt and serve.

Vegetarian Option: Substitute the prawns with 60g (1/2 cup) marinated tofu pieces instead. Calories per serving 195

Serves: 2   Ready In: 10 mins   Per Serving: 167 Calories

Baked Eggs with Roasted Asparagus & Parma Ham

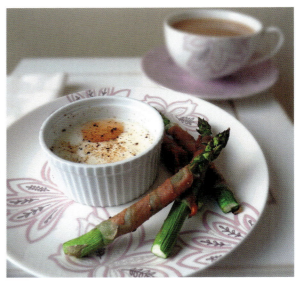

Ingredients
- 8 fresh, medium asparagus spears –22 cals
- 4 slices Parma ham, all fat removed –35 cals
- 2 UK med (US Large) free range eggs –88 cals
- 2 tbsp half-fat sour cream –18 cals
- 4 sprays of Frylight olive oil spray –2 cals
- pinch sea (kosher) salt
- pinch freshly ground black pepper
- pinch freshly grated nutmeg

Directions
Preheat the oven to 180C fan, 350F, Gas Mark 6.

Spritz two oven-proof ramekins with a spray of Frylight olive oil spray and place on a baking tray. Break the eggs into the ramekin, then spoon a tbsp of sour cream over each egg. Season with a pinch of salt and a light grating of nutmeg. Pop into the oven.

Meanwhile, trim the woody ends off the asparagus spears. Trim all visible fat from the slices of Parma ham and cut in half. Wrap each asparagus spear with a ½ slice of ham. After the eggs have been in the oven for 7 mins (or 10 mins if you prefer firmly cooked eggs), spread the Parma-wrapped asparagus spears onto the baking sheet, season with freshly ground black pepper and spritz with 2 sprays of olive oil spray. Return the baking sheet to the oven and cook for a further 8 mins (so that the eggs will cook for 15-18 mins in total). Once cooked, remove from the oven and transfer to warm plates to serve.

Serves: 2   Ready In: 15 mins   Per Serving: 166 Calories

Mediterranean Cous Cous Salad (V)

Ingredients with cals per serving

- 55g ($^1/_3$ cup) cous cous (dry weight) – 103 cals
- 1 orange bell pepper –25 cals
- artichoke hearts –15 cals (tinned or frozen, not oil 88g)
- 4 cherry tomatoes (45g) –6 cals
- black olives, drained (13g) –11 cals
- 4 large spring onions/scallions (80g) - 10 cals
- ¼ English cucumber (45g) –4 cals
- 15g (1½ tbsp) raisins –11 cals
- 1 tbsp fresh basil, chopped –1 cal
- 1 tbsp fresh parsley, chopped –1 cal
- ½ vegetable stock cube –8 cals
- ½ lemon, juiced –2 cals
- pinch saffron
- pinch ground black pepper
- pinch sea (kosher) salt

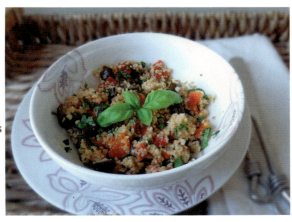

Directions

In a microwave proof jug, dissolve ½ stock cube in 85mls of boiling water and add the pinch of saffron. Allow to infuse for 10 mins. Pour the dry cous cous into a heat proof bowl. Reheat the water to close to boiling point in the microwave on high for 1 min, pour over the cous cous and cover the bowl with cling wrap. Set aside for 5 mins whilst you prepare the salad vegetables.

Slice the pepper and artichoke hearts into bite-size pieces. Halve the cherry tomatoes and olives. Slice the spring onions. Peel and deseed the cucumber and cube the flesh. Finely chop the basil and parsley.

After 5 mins, remove the cling wrap form the bowl of cous cous. Fluff up the cous cous with a fork, season with salt and pepper and add the lemon juice and chopped herbs. Mix well. Add the salad vegetables and toss. Divide between 2 plates and serve.

Serves: 2   Ready In: 25 mins   Per Serving: 197 Calories

Two-Day 5:2 Diet Dinners
5:2 Diet Dinners 200 Calories & Under

Courgette & Chickpea Balti (V)

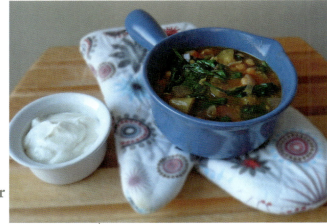

Ingredients with cals per serving

- 1 red onion 80g –16 cals
- 1 medium courgettes (zucchini) 300g (1½ cups) –30 cals–7 cals
- 120g (½ cup + 1 tbsp) canned, drained chickpeas - 68 cals
- 20g (3 tbsp) fresh root ginger, grated –4 cals
- 1 tbsp balti paste –23 cals
- 90g (3 cups) baby spinach –14 cals
- 2 medium tomatoes 160g - 16 cals
- ½ reduced salt vegetable stock cube
- ½ lime –5 cals
- 2 tbsp 0% fat Greek yogurt –9 cals
- 2 sprays Frylight olive oil spray
- 2 garlic cloves –4 cals
- pinch black pepper and sea salt

Directions

Skin the tomatoes by placing in a bowl and covering with boiling water. Leave for 1 min, then carefully remove from the water with a slotted spoon. Peel and discard the skin. Roughly cop the tomatoes and set aside. Finely dice the onion and slice the courgette/zucchini. Heat a sauté pan with a lid over a medium heat and spritz with 2 sprays of Frylight olive oil spray. Add the courgette/zucchini and onions and sauté for 5 mins until golden. Meanwhile, dissolve the ½ stock cube in 120ml (½ cup) of boiling water. Finely mince the garlic and grate the ginger. Add these to the sauté pan and fry for a further minute. Stir in the chopped tomatoes and balti curry paste. Add the chickpeas and vegetable stock and stir. Cover with the pan lid and simmer for 10 mins. Finally, juice the ½ lime and add this to the curry along with the baby spinach, salt and pepper. Stir until the spinach wilts. Serve with Greek yogurt on the side.

Want to Add Rice? 60g (½ cup) dry Brown Basmati Rice between two people adds 113 calories per person.

Serves: 2   **Ready In:** 35 mins   **Per Serving:** 195 Calories

Sweet & Sour Chicken

Ingredients with cals per serving
- 120g (4 oz) skinless chicken breast –64 cals
- 1 red bell pepper –25 cals
- 4 small spring onions/scallions –3 cals
- 216g (1 cup) tinned pineapple chunks in juice (½ tin) –57 cals
- 50g (½ cup) chestnut (baby portabella) mushrooms –4 cals
- 100g (1 cup) beansprouts (mung) –17 cals
- 1 tsp light brown sugar –10 cals
- ½ tbsp cornflour (corn starch) –7 cals
- 2 tbsp rice wine vinegar –3 cals
- 1 garlic clove –2 cals
- 1 fresh red chilli (10g) –3 cals
- sprays Frylight olive oil spray –1 cals
- 1 tbsp light soy sauce –7 cals
- pinch ground black pepper
- pinch sea (kosher) salt

Directions

Deseed and slice the red chilli and pepper. Slice the spring onions (scallions), mushrooms and garlic clove. Cut the chicken breast into bite size pieces. Put the cornflour (corn starch) and brown sugar into a jug and dissolve with 2 tbsp of juice from the canned pineapple. Heat a wok over a medium heat and spritz with 2 sprays of Frylight olive oil spray. Add the pepper and onions and stir-fry for 3-4 mins. Add the chicken pieces, red chilli and garlic and stir-fry until the chicken is lightly golden.

Meanwhile, heat a separate non-stick sauté pan over a medium heat and dry fry the slice mushrooms. When the chicken is lightly golden, add the pineapple chunks and their juice. Stir the corn starch/sugar mixture thoroughly to ensure that it is fully dissolved and add to the pan. Bring to a light simmer and season with salt and pepper.

Add the beansprouts to the dry-fried mushrooms and sauté whilst the chicken mixture finishes cooking. Check that the chicken pieces are cooked through, then divide the mushrooms and beansprouts between two plates and then spoon over the sweet and sour chicken to serve.

Vegetarian Option: Substitute the chicken breast with Quorn chicken style fillet instead. Calories per serving 188

Want to Add Rice? 60g (½ cup) dried weight of brown basmati rice between two people adds 113 calories per person

Serves: 2   Ready In: 20 mins   Per Serving: 200 Calories

Black Bean Pepper Hash (V)

Ingredients with cals per serving
- 200g (7 oz) new potatoes (Charlotte or Yukon gold) –75 cals
- 1 medium shallot (50g) –12 cals
- 1 yellow bell pepper –25 cals
- 150g (1½ cups) chestnut (baby portabella) mushrooms –12 cals
- 2 medium tomatoes –13 cals
- 60g (⅓ cup) dried black beans –57 cals
- dash Tabasco
- 1 garlic clove, minced –2 cals
- ½ tsp ground cumin –1 cal
- ½ tsp dried red chilli flakes –1 cal
- ½ tsp dried oregano
- 2 tbsp fresh coriander/cilantro, chopped –1 cal
- 2 sprays Frylight olive oil spray –1 cal
- pinch ground black pepper and sea (kosher) salt

Directions

Overnight, place the dried black beans into sealable container, cover with fresh water and leave to soak overnight. When ready to start on the meal, drain and rinse the beans, place in a saucepan with 350mls (1½ cups) of fresh water. Bring to the boil and boil rapidly, uncovered for 10 mins, then reduce the heat, cover the pan and simmer for a further 30 mins. Drain and rinse. Alternatively, substitute the 60g (⅓ cup) of dried black beans for 135g (½ cup) canned black beans, drained and well rinsed.

Cut (but don't peel) the potatoes into bite sized chunks. Place in a saucepan, cover with cold water and a pinch of salt. Bring to the boil and simmer until tender (5-10 mins, depending on how large your pieces are).

Meanwhile, deseed and slice the pepper. Clean and thickly slice the mushrooms. Cut the shallot in half length-wise and thinly slice. Mince the garlic cloves. Heat a non-stick sauté pan over a medium heat and spritz with 2 sprays of Frylight olive oil spray. Add the shallots and stir-fry for 3-4 mins. Drain the potatoes well and add these to the non-stick sauté pan along with mushrooms and sliced peppers. Continue to sauté.

Dice the tomatoes and chop the fresh coriander (cilantro). Once the sautéed potatoes have turned a lovely golden brown, add the rinsed, cooked black beans, diced tomatoes, coriander (cilantro) and the herbs and spices. Add as many dashes of Tabasco (hot chilli) sauce as suits your tastes. Season with a pinch of freshly ground pepper and salt. Continue to turn the hash in the non-stick sauté pan until the beans and tomatoes are completely warmed through, then divide between 2 dinner plates and serve.

Serves: 2 Ready In: 40 mins (plus soaking time) **Per Serving: 199 Calories**

Garlic & Herb Roasted Cod with Fennel En Papillote

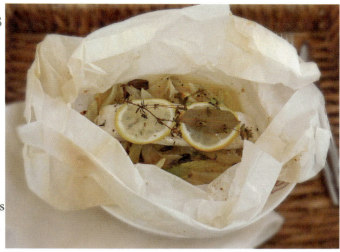

Ingredients with cals per serving

- 250g (9 oz) sustainably-caught cod fillets −100 cals
- 260g (3 cups) fennel bulb, sliced − 41 cals
- 1 lemon −6 cals
- 6 pitted green olives in brine (15g) −15 cals
- 6 stalks fresh flat-leaf parsley −2 cals
- 2 sprays Frylight olive oil spray −1 cal
- 6 sprigs fresh thyme −2 cals
- 1 garlic clove, minced −1 cals
- 2 bay leaves
- pinch black pepper and sea salt

Directions

Preheat the oven to 180C fan, 375F, Gas Mark 6. Slice the fennel into thin-ish slices, halve the olives and place both in a bowl. Set aside 2 springs of thyme, then remove the leaves from the remaining sprigs and finely chop these along with the flat-leaf parsley. Sprinkle half of these chopped herbs over the fennel and olives. Mince the garlic and add this to bowl. Cut the lemon in half, slice one half and set aside. Juice the other half and add this to the fennel/olives. Finally, season with salt and pepper, and toss well. Take 2 pieces of parchment paper, each 30cmx45cm (12"x18"). Place the sheets onto a baking sheet. Divide the seasoned fennel slices even onto the 2 sheets. Place a fish fillet on top each of the piles of fennel and sprinkle it with the remaining chopped herbs and season with salt and pepper. Divide the lemon slices between the 2 pieces of cod, then top with a sprig of thyme, a bay leaf and a spray of Frylight. To seal each parcel, bring the parchment over the fish, join together the long edges and fold over to seal. Double-fold each end and tuck under to make a sealed parcel. (see right) The parcel should not be too tight, as steam will puff it up in the oven, but the edges need to be sealed to prevent steam & liquid escaping whilst cooking. Place the baking sheet in the oven and cook for 15 mins. Remove from oven and allow to rest for 2 mins. Then to serve, place a papillote on a warm dinner plate. Then simply cut open the papillote and eat the contents inside.

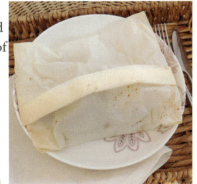

Serves: 2   **Ready In:** 40 mins   **Per Serving:** 199 Calories

Indonesian Chicken with Asian Slaw

Ingredients with cals per serving

- 170g (6 oz) skinless chicken breast - 91
- 2 tsp clear honey –17 cals
- 2 tbsp dark soy sauce –9 cals
- 1½ tbsp grated ginger, divided –6 cals
- 2 garlic cloves, minced –4 cals
- 50g (²/₃ cup) shredded red cabbage –8 cals
- 50g (¹/₃ cup) raw celeriac/jicama –5 cals
- 1 medium carrot (60g), grated –12 cals
- ½ lime, juiced –5 cal
- 2 tbsp fresh coriander/cilantro –2 cals
- 1 tsp toasted sesame seeds –8 cals
- ½ tbsp rice wine vinegar
- ½ tsp toasted sesame oil –10 cals
- ¹/₃ tsp soft brown sugar - 10 cals
- ½ fresh red chilli –1 cal
- pinch black pepper and sea salt

Directions

If possible, make the marinade (below) in the morning and put the chicken and marinade in a sealed container in the fridge until cooking in the evening.

Preheat the oven to 160C fan, 350F, Gas Mark 6.

In a bowl, mix together the honey, soy sauce, minced garlic and 1 tbsp of grated ginger. Cut the chicken breast into 2 even pieces and place in a cast-iron lidded casserole dish (Dutch oven). Pour over the marinade. Make sure that the lid to the casserole fits tightly, if not, cover the casserole dish (Dutch oven) with tightly fitted aluminium foil. Place into oven and roast chicken for 25 mins until cooked through.

Deseed and mince the red chilli and pepper. Chop the coriander (cilantro), grate the carrot and shred the cabbage and celeriac (jicama). In a bowl, whisk together the retained ½ tbsp of grated ginger, Rice Wine Vinegar, toasted sesame oil, lime juice, brown sugar, salt and pepper. Add a dash of Tabasco sauce, if you like a real kick to your slaw. Add the shredded slaw vegetables and toss together.

If you have only been able to source raw sesame seeds, then dry-roast the seeds in a non-stick sauté pan over a medium heat. Keep tossing the seeds and watch them like a hawk. Remove from pan as soon as seeds are toasted and scatter over the slaw.

Divide the slaw between two dinner plates. Remove the chicken from the oven once cooked and divide between the plates. Spoon any cooking juices over the chicken and serve.

Vegetarian Option: Substitute the chicken breast with Quorn chicken style fillet instead. Calories per serving 168

Want to Add Noodles? 150g/5 oz packet of Straight to Wok Rice Noodles divided between two people adds 97 calories per portion

Serves: 2   Ready In: 30 mins   Per Serving: 186 Calories

Tandoori Chicken Kebabs

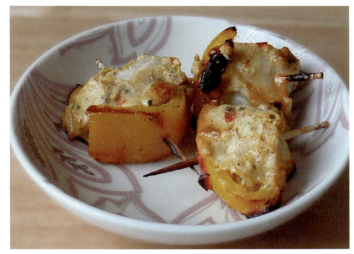

Note: If possible, make the marinade (below) in the morning and put the chicken and marinade in a sealed container in the fridge until cooking in the evening.

Ingredients with cals per serving

- 140g (5 oz) skinless chicken breast –87 cals
- 1 yellow bell pepper –25 cals
- ½ lime, juiced –5 cals
- 1½ tbsp grated fresh ginger, divided –6 cals
- 2 garlic cloves, minced –4 cals
- 120g (½ cup) 0% fat Greek yogurt –34 cals
- 90g (3 cups) baby leaf salad –16 cals
- 1 tsp paprika –3 cal
- ½ tsp ground coriander –1 cals
- 1 fresh red chilli, minced –3 cals
- ½ lime, juiced –5 cals
- ½ tsp ground cumin –1 cals
- 1 tsp garam masala –2 cals
- pinch ground turmeric
- pinch ground black pepper
- pinch sea (kosher) salt

Directions

Deseed and mince the red chilli, along with the garlic. Grate the ginger. In a bowl, mix together the ginger, garlic, yogurt, lime juice, chilli, spices, salt and pepper. Cut the chicken breast into even bite size pieces and mix into the marinade. Cover and leave to marinade for 30 mins or longer in the fridge. Meanwhile, if using wooden or bamboo skewers, soak in water to prevent scorching whilst cooking.

Preheat the oven to 180C fan, 350F, Gas Mark 6. Preheat a non-stick baking tray. Chop the yellow pepper into even sized pieces. Thread onto the skewer, alternating with the chicken pieces. Place the skewers onto the heated baking tray and bake in the oven for 20 mins or until the chicken pieces are completely cooked through. Divide the baby leaf salad between two dinner plates. Remove the skewers from the oven once cooked and divide between the plates.

Vegetarian Option: Substitute the chicken breast with Quorn chicken style fillet instead. Calories per serving 166

Want to Add Rice? 60g (½ cup) dried weight of brown basmati rice between two people adds 113 calories per person

Serves: 2   Ready In: 25 mins   Per Serving: 190 Calories

Ragout of Lamb & Beans

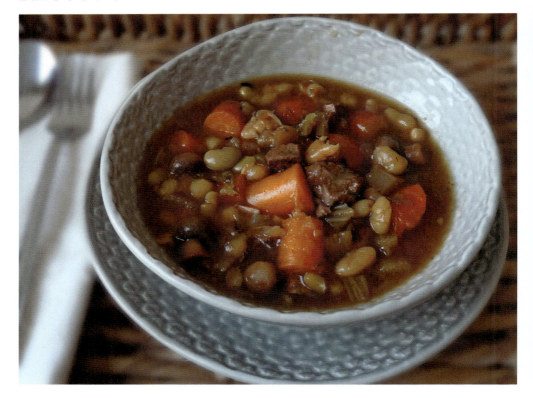

Ingredients with cals per serving

- 110g (4 oz) lean lamb leg steaks, all visible fat removed –66 cals
- 100g (¾ cup) Chantenay carrots (or 8 baby carrots), trimmed –20 cals
- 1 stick of celery heart –1 cals
- 8 cherry tomatoes –10 cals
- 1 garlic clove, minced –2 cals
- 150g (5 oz) button (baby bella) mushrooms –12 cals
- 1 medium red onion (c 80g) –16 cals
- 132g (4½ oz) tinned flageolet beans, drained –47 cals
- 2 sprays Frylight olive oil spray –1 cal
- 8g (1 tbsp) cornflour (corn starch) –14 cal
- 5-6 sprigs fresh thyme –2 cals
- 2 bay leaves
- ½ lamb stock cube –8 cal
- pinch ground black pepper
- pinch sea (kosher) salt

Note: You may want to make double of this recipe and freeze half, as it does freeze beautifully and then makes a quick and easy 5:2 dinner to have to hand.

Directions

Preheat the oven to 140C fan, 275F, Gas Mark 1. Alternatively, this can be cooked in a slow cooker/crockpot.

Drain the tinned flageolet and rinse thoroughly. Set aside. Put the cherry tomatoes into a heat proof jug and pour over enough boiling water to cover generously. Wait 30 secs, then carefully drain away the hot water. De-skin the tomatoes and set aside. In the jug, dissolve the lamb stock cube in 240ml (1 cup) of boiling water.

Trim all visible fat from the lamb leg steaks and cut into bite size pieces. Heat a non-stick sauté pan over a medium heat and spritz with 2 sprays of Frylight olive oil spray. Add the lamb pieces to the pan and brown on all sides until the meat is golden and slightly caramelised. Remove from the pan and keep to one side.

Meanwhile, dice the onion and celery. Once the meat has been removed from the pan, sauté the onions and celery until translucent (3-4) mins. Clean the button mushrooms and add these to the non-stick sauté pan. After 3-4 mins, add the minced garlic and fry for a further 1 min. Cut the carrots in half length-wise. Pour over the stock, and return the lamb to the pan, along with the tomatoes, drained beans and halved carrots.

Rinse the jug out with cold water to cool it down, then dissolve the cornflour (corn starch) in 2 tablespoons of cold water. Add to the stew, and bring the mixture to the simmer, stirring all the time until the sauce thickens. Season with salt and pepper and transfer all of the ingredients to a heavy casserole dish (Dutch oven) or slow cooker pot (if using). Tuck the sprigs of thyme and bay leaves into the stew. Cover with a lid.

Cook the stew in the low oven or slow cooker for 2.5 hrs until tender and flavoursome. Divide between 2 warmed dinner plates and serve.

Serves: 2   Ready In: 2 hrs 30 mins   Per Serving: 200 Calories

Aromatic Duck with Plum Sauce & Sautéed Cabbage

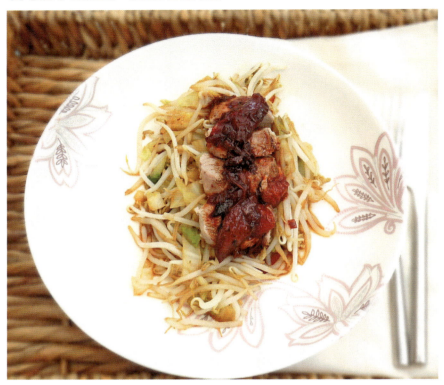

Ingredients with cals per serving

- 170g (6 oz) skinless duck breast −78 cals
- 1 shallot (40g) −4 cal
- 2 tbsp red wine −11 cal
- 3 plums (medium) −46 cal
- 1 tsp light brown sugar −9 cal
- 1 tsp Chinese 5 spice powder −1 cal
- 2 tsp dark soy sauce (divided) −6 cal
- 2 garlic cloves (divided) −4 cal
- ½ star anise −2 cal
- 150g (2 cups) savoy cabbage, shredded −20 cals
- 50g (½ cup) beansprouts (mung) −9 cal
- ½ chicken stock cube −8 cal
- 3 sprays Frylight olive oil spray −1 cal
- pinch ground black pepper
- pinch sea (kosher) salt

Tip 1: Buy a small bottle of red wine and decant 1 tablespoon servings into an ice-cube tray. Freeze and use as required in cooking.

Tip 2: If you can, prepare the sauce and marinate the duck in advance to allow the flavours to develop fully.

Directions

Remove any skin he duck breast. Finely mince 1 garlic clove. In a sealable container, whisk together the minced garlic clove, the Chinese 5 spice powder, a good pinch of ground black pepper and 1 tsp of dark soy sauce. Add the duck breast and turn it over in the marinade several times to ensure that it is well coated. Seal the container and put in the fridge to marinade for at least 30 mins but preferably several hours. If you are able to also prepare the Plum Sauce too in advance, do this now and set aside (see below).

Preheat the oven to 180C fan, 375F, Gas Mark 6. Heat a non-stick sauté pan over a medium-high heat and spritz with a spray of Frylight olive oil spray. Add the duck breast and cook 2 minutes on each side. Transfer to a roasting dish and roast for 8-10 minutes. Remove the duck breast from the oven, cover with aluminium foil and rest for 10 mins.

Meanwhile, finely chop the shallot and divide into 2 portions. Halve the plums and remove the stones. Cut each half into thirds. In a jug, dissolve the stock cube in 120ml ($1/2$ cup) boiling water. Set aside 20ml (4 tsps) of the stock.

Heat a small non-stick saucepan over a medium heat and spritz with a spray of Frylight spray. Add half of the chopped shallot to the pan and sauté for 3-4 mins until softened. Add the wine and allow it to bubble up, then add the plums, sugar, star anise and the 100ml chicken stock. Simmer for 10 mins until reduced and thickened. Set aside.

Whilst the duck breast rests, reheat the sauté pan and spritz with a spray of Frylight. Add the remaining chopped shallot to the pan and sauté 3-4 minutes until soft, then add the remaining minced garlic and cook for a further minute. Add the shredded cabbage and toss. Stir fry for 2-3 mins then add the retained 20ml (4 tsps) of the stock and the remaining tsp of soy sauce. Season with salt and black pepper and simmer for 2-3 mins until cooked through.

Divide the sautéed cabbage between 2 warm dinner plates. Slice the duck breast into 6-8 slices and place 3-4 on each plate. Spoon over the plum sauce and serve.

Want to Add Noodles? 150g/5 oz of cooked Rice Noodles divided between two people adds 97 calories per portion

Serves: 2   Ready In: 20 mins (plus marinating time)   Per Serving: 199 Calories

5:2 Dinners 300 Calories & Under

Mushroom Stroganoff with Basmati Rice (V)

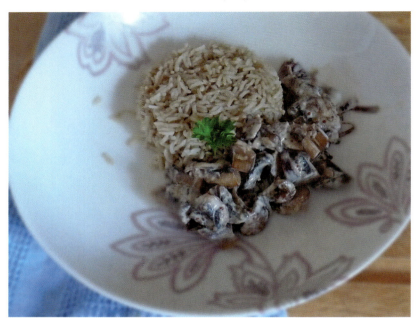

Ingredients with cals per serving

- 250g (2½ cup) chestnut (baby portabella) mushrooms –20 cal
- 10g (1 tbsp) mixed dried mushrooms –13 cals
- 1 medium shallot –5 cals
- 2 garlic cloves –5 cals
- 1 tsp dried thyme –2 cals
- 1 tsp cornflour/corn starch –6 cals
- ½ beef stock cube –4 cals
- ½ tbsp Dijon mustard –6 cals
- 2 tbsp Madeira wine –21 cals
- 2 tbsp half fat crème fraîche –28 cals
- 25g (2 scant tbsp) 3% fat soft cheese –29 cals
- 2 sprays Frylight olive oil spray –1 cal
- 1 tbsp mushroom ketchup (optional, see note) –11 cals
- pinch ground black pepper
- pinch sea (kosher) salt
- 60g (½ cup) brown basmati rice, dried weight –113 cals

Note: Geo Watkins Mushroom Ketchup is a wonderful savoury sauce, it's found in the speciality food section of good supermarkets and will add a rich, savoury flavour to your cooking. If you can't (or don't want to) find it, you can substitute Worcestershire Sauce instead.

Directions

In a jug, dissolve the ½ beef stock cube in 100ml boiling water. Add the dried mushrooms, set aside and leave to soak.

Put the basmati rice into a saucepan with twice the quantity of cold water and a pinch of salt. Bring to the boil and cook for 20 mins.

Clean and slice the chestnut (baby portabella) mushrooms. Cut the shallot in half length-wise and thinly slice. Mince the garlic cloves. Heat a non-stick sauté pan over a medium heat and spritz with 2 sprays of Frylight olive oil spray. Add the shallots and stir-fry for 3-4 mins. Add the chestnut (baby portabella) mushrooms and continue to sauté.

Meanwhile, in a jug, mix together the crème fraîche, soft cheese, mustard and cornflour(corn starch). When fully combined, slacken with the Madeira wine and mushroom ketchup (if using).

Remove the dried mushrooms from the stock, reserving the steeping liquid. Slice the mushrooms into small pieces. Add these and the garlic to the non-stick sauté pan and cook for 1 min. Carefully pour in the reserved steeping liquid, taking care to not add any grit that may have come out of the dried mushrooms. Stir the crème/wine/cornflour (corn starch) mixture again to ensure it is still dissolved then add this to the pan. Stir until the mixture has come to the boil and thickened. Season and cook for a further minute. Drain the rice and divide between 2 warmed plates. Spoon over the Mushroom Stroganoff.

Serves: 2   Ready In: 25 mins   Per Serving: 271 Calories

Choucroute Garni with Mustard Cream Sauce

Ingredients with cals per serving

- 2 low fat chicken sausages (95 cals each eg Marks & Spencer) –95 cals
- 70g (2½ oz) reduced fat smoked pork sausage –84 cals
- ½ medium white onion, chopped (2 tbsp) –12 cals
- 1 garlic clove, minced –2 cals
- 225g (1½ cup) sauerkraut, drained and rinsed –21 cal
- 2 tbsp apple juice (apple cider) –7 cal
- 60ml (¼ cup) dry white wine –22 cal
- ¼ tsp ground allspice
- ½ tsp caraway seeds –2 cals
- 2 sprays Frylight olive oil spray –1 cal
- pinch ground black pepper
- 2 tbsp half fat sour cream –18 cals
- 1 tbsp Dijon mustard –12 cals

Directions

Preheat the oven to 180C fan, 375F, Gas Mark 6.

Thoroughly rinse the sauerkraut and leave to drain.

Heat a flame-proof casserole dish (Dutch oven) over a medium heat. When hot, spritz with 2 sprays of Frylight olive oil spray then add the chicken sausages and brown on all sides. Thickly slice the smoked pork sausage and sauté with the chicken sausage. Chop the onion. Remove the meat and set to one side. Add the onion to the hot casserole and sauté until translucent, about 5 minutes. Mince the garlic and add to the onion, cook for a further minute. Add drained sauerkraut, apple juice, white wine, allspice and caraway seeds. Bring up to a simmer. Slice the chicken sausages in half, then return all the sausage meat to the casserole, nestling them amongst the sauerkraut mixture. Season with black pepper. Put the lid on the casserole and bake in the oven for 30 mins.

Whilst the choucroute is cooking, whisk together the sour cream and Dijon mustard and chill.

When baked, divide the casserole between 2 warm dinner plates and serve with the chilled mustard sour cream.

Want to Add Potatoes? 225g (3 cups) of steamed new potatoes divided between two people adds 86 calories per portion.

Serves: 2   Ready In: 45 mins   Per Serving: 279 Calories

Tuna Niçoise Salad

Ingredients with cals per serving

- 200g (7 oz) fresh tuna steaks –136 cals
- 140g (5 oz) new potatoes (Charlotte or Yukon gold) –52 cals
- 100g (½ cup) trimmed green beans –15 cals
- 4 cherry tomatoes (45g) –6 cals
- 4 black olives, drained (10g) –10 cals
- 2 anchovy fillets –4 cals
- 1 UK med (US large) free range egg –44 cals
- 1 baby gem lettuce head –8 cals
- 2 tsp Dijon mustard - 8 cals
- 2 tbsp white wine vinegar –3 cals
- 2 tbsp fresh parsley, chopped –1 cal
- 2 tbsp fresh basil, shredded –1 cal
- 2 sprays Frylight olive oil –1 cal
- pinch ground black pepper
- pinch sea (kosher) salt

Directions

Hard boil the egg by placing the room temperature egg in a pan of cold water, bring up to simmering point and then simmer for 7 minutes. As soon as the egg is cooked, drain off the hot water, then plunge the egg into plenty of cold water for one minute. Then drain again and cover with more fresh cold water. Leave for about 2 mins until cool enough to handle and then shell and set to one side.

Cut each of the new potatoes (skin on) into quarters length-wise. Bring a pan of salted water to the boil and add the potato quarters. Cook until tender (5-8 mins, dependent on size), then remove from pan with a slotted spoon and set aside. Bring the water back up to the boil and quickly blanch the trimmed green beans (cook for 2-3 mins until tender but still crisp). Drain and plunge the cooked beans into a bowl of iced water to cool quickly. Once cooled, drain on kitchen towel.

In a bowl, whisk together the mustard, vinegar and chopped herbs. Finely chop the anchovy fillets and add to the vinaigrette. Halve the cherry tomatoes and quarter the olives and add these to the vinaigrette along with the cooled potatoes and green beans. Toss together well.

Heat a non-stick sauté pan over a medium heat and spritz with 2 sprays of Frylight olive oil spray. Cook the tuna steaks for 2-3 minutes on each side, depending on how rare you like your fish.

Separate the lettuce leaves, rinse, drain and dry them. Divide them between 2 dinner plates and spoon over the dressed vegetables. Cut the boiled egg in half and then cut each half into three portions. Scatter over the salad then top with the cooked and sliced tuna steak.

Vegetarian Option: Substitute the tuna steaks with 120g (1 cup) marinated tofu pieces instead and omit the anchovy fillets. Calories per serving 281

Serves: 2 **Ready In:** 25 mins **Per Serving:** 284 Calories

Individual Cottage Pies (V)

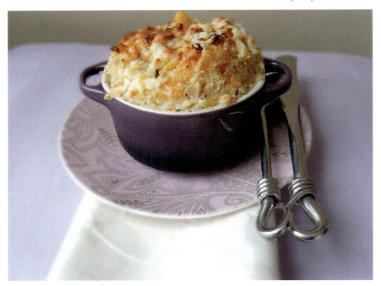

Ingredients

- 30g ($^1/_6$ cup) dried green lentils –14 cals
- 30g ($^1/_6$ cup) dried yellow split peas –15 cals
- 30g ($^1/_6$ cup) dried white beans (cannellini or great northern) –17 cals
- 1 medium courgette (zucchini) 200g (1½ cups) –10 cals
- 1 red pepper –13 cals
- 2 medium carrots 120g (1 cup) –11 cals
- 150g (1½ cups) butternut squash (peeled and deseeded weight) –16 cals
- 150g (1½ cups) fennel –11 cals
- 1 red onion (80g) –8 cals
- 240g (2 cups) chestnut (baby portabella) mushrooms –10 cals
- 2 tsp mixed herbs –2 cals
- 2 garlic cloves –2 cals
- ½ tsp chilli pepper flakes –1 cal
- 1 reduced salt vegetable stock cube –8 cals
- 2 medium tomatoes –8 cals
- 10g (2 tsp) cornflour (corn starch) –7 cals
- 450g (3 cups) swede (rutabaga), peeled and diced - 33
- 2 parsnips 230g (1 cup), peeled and diced - 44
- 28g (2 tbsp) 3% fat soft cheese –8 cals
- 28g (2 tbsp) half fat mature cheese, grated –19 cals
- 2 sprays Frylight olive oil spray
- ground black pepper and sea (kosher) salt, divided

Directions

You will need to pre-soak the white beans in 240ml (½ cup) of cold water overnight. After soaking, drain the beans then give them a good rinse them along with lentils and split peas. Put the drained beans, split peas and lentils into a saucepan. Add 500ml (2 cups) of cold water, cover and simmer gently for 30 mins. If you have forgotten to soak the beans, you can use canned beans, instead. In this case, use 70g ($^1/_3$ cup), rinse thoroughly and add to the lentils and peas after they have cooked. Drain and set aside.

Meanwhile, peel and dice the swede (rutabaga) parsnips into big chunks and place in a saucepan, cover with cold water and add a pinch of salt. Bring up to the boil and simmer for 15 mins. Add the parsnips and continue to simmer until tender (about another 10 mins). When cooked, drain and return to the saucepan and mash. Then whisk in the soft cheese to form a rustic purée and set aside until needed.

Meanwhile, prepare the butternut squash by first peeling, then use a spoon to remove and discard the fibrous centre and seeds. De-seed the pepper too. Cut the peppers, courgette (zucchini), carrots and squash into 2.5cm (1") cubes. Preheat the oven to 180C fan, 400F, Gas Mark 6.

Dice the red onion and fennel. Heat a sauté pan over a medium heat and spritz with 2 sprays of Frylight olive oil spray. Add the onion and fennel to the pan and sauté for 5 minutes until softened, stirring occasionally. Add the red peppers, courgette (zucchini), squash and carrots. Cook for 3-4 mins. Slice the mushrooms and add these to the pan, cook for a further 5 mins. Finely mince the garlic cloves and add to the vegetables and cook for 1 min. In a jug, dissolve vegetable stock cube in 240ml (1 cup) of boiling water. Add to the vegetables. Dissolve the cornflour (corn starch) in 2 tbsp of cold water and stir into the vegetable stew. Keep stirring and bring up to a gentle simmer, until slightly thickened (about 1 min). Remove from the heat and stir in the drained beans, mixed herbs, red chilli flakes and ¼ tsp ground black pepper. Mix well. Divide the bean and vegetable stew between 4 oven-proof ramekins. Slice the tomatoes and divide over the top of the bean stew. Finally, spread over the mashed swede and parsnip and sprinkle with the grated mature cheese.

Pop the Cottage Pies onto a baking sheet and cook on the top shelf of the preheated oven for 20-25 mins, or until the top is lightly browned and the pies are piping hot.

Cooking for 1 or 2? Prepare & Freeze Meal Tip:

Once the pies are assembled (but before baking), allow to cool, then seal with kitchen foil and freeze. To cook, defrost, remove kitchen foil and then bake in a preheated oven (180C fan, 400F, Gas Mark 6) for 25-30 mins until piping hot and golden.

Want to Add Potatoes? 225g (3 cups) of steamed new potatoes divided between two people adds 86 calories per portion.

Serves: 4   Ready In: 1 hr 15 mins   Per Serving: 250 Calories

Parma-Wrapped Chicken & Garlicky Roast Potatoes

Ingredients with cals per serving

- 250g (9 oz) skinless chicken breast fillets –155 cals
- 140g (5 oz) new potatoes (Charlotte or Yukon gold) –52 cals
- 2 thin slices Parma ham (fat removed) –20 cals
- 6 sage leaves –2 cals
- 45g (3 tbsp) 3% fat soft cheese –25 cals
- 2 garlic cloves, minced –3 cals
- 2 sprays Frylight olive oil spray –1 cal
- 100g (½ cup) trimmed green beans –15 cal
- pinch ground black pepper
- pinch sea (kosher) salt

Directions

Preheat the oven to 180C fan, 375F, Gas Mark 6. Place a roasting tin in the oven to heat through.

Cut the potatoes (skin on) into half. Bring a pan of salted water to the boil and add the potatoes. Par-boil for 5 mins.

Meanwhile, finely chop the garlic and divide into 2 halves. Remove the stalks from the sage leaves and shred. In a bowl, mix together the soft cheese, half the garlic and all of the sage. Season with salt and pepper. Using a sharp knife, cut a slit along each chicken breast to make a pocket. Divide the cheese mixture between each breast. Fold the chicken back into shape and wrap each breast in a slice of Parma ham.

Drain the par-boiled potatoes. Remove the roasting tin from the oven, add the drained potatoes, sprinkle with the reserved minced garlic and spritz with 2 sprays of Frylight olive oil spray. Toss together to ensure the potatoes are evenly coated with the oil and garlic. Nestle the 2 Parma-wrapped chicken breasts amongst the potatoes. Return to the oven and bake in the oven for 25-30 minutes until cooked through.

Just before serving, steam the green beans for 3-4 mins, then divide between 2 warm dinner plates. Remove the cooked chicken breasts and potatoes to the dinner plates and spoon over any juices from the roasting pan. Serve.

Serves: 2   Ready In: 35 mins   Per Serving: 273 Calories

Creamy Mustard Pork

Ingredients with cals per serving

- 110g (4 oz) lean pork escalope –88 cals
- 120g (4 oz) button (baby bella) mushrooms –10 cals
- 1 medium shallot (50g) –12 cals
- 1 garlic cloves –2 cals
- ½ vegetable stock cube –8 cals
- ½ tbsp Dijon mustard –6 cals
- ½ tbsp wholegrain mustard –7 cals
- ½ tsp dry mustard powder –4 cals
- 2 tbsp half fat crème fraîche –28 cals
- 25g (2 scant tbsp) 3% fat soft cheese –29 cals
- 2 sprays Frylight olive oil spray –1 cal
- pinch ground black pepper and sea (kosher) salt
- 60g (½ cup) whole-wheat pasta, dry weight –102 cals

Directions

Remove any fat from the pork escalope and cut into strips. Clean the mushrooms and slice them too. Finely chop the garlic. Cut the shallot in half length-wise and then slice into thin slices.

In a small bowl, mix together the three mustards with the crème fraîche and soft cheese. In a heat-proof jug, dissolve the stock cube into 60ml (¼ cup) boiling water.

Put the dry pasta in a saucepan, cover with plenty of cold water and a pinch of salt and bring to the boil. Simmer until cooked, according to the packet instructions.

Heat a non-stick sauté pan over a medium heat and spritz with 2 sprays of Frylight olive oil spray. Add the shallot and stir-fry gently for about 2-3 minutes until softened. Add the sliced mushrooms to the pan, continue to sauté for 4 mins until lightly cooked. Add the garlic and cook for a further minute then remove everything from the pan onto a plate and set aside.

Turn the heat up under the pan to high and heat through, then add the pork and stir-fry quickly, until the pork is lightly golden. Return the reserved vegetables to the pan and warm through. Add the stock and let it bubble and reduce slightly before adding the crème fraîche/mustard mixture. Let the sauce bubble and reduce to half its original volume. Season to taste with salt and pepper. Drain the cooked pasta and divide between 2 warm serving plates. Spoon over the creamy mustard pork and serve.

Vegetarian Option: Substitute the pork with 110g (1 cup) tofu pieces instead. Calories per serving 252.

Serves: 2   Ready In: 25 mins   Per Serving: 298 Calories

GRILLED SEA BASS WITH SALSA VERDE

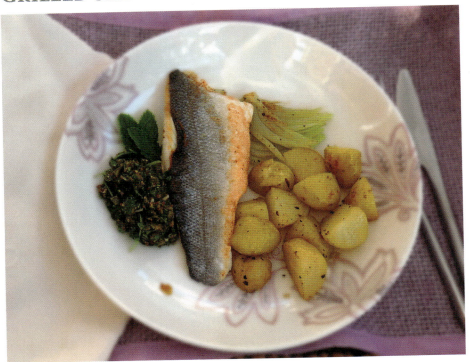

Ingredients with cals per serving

- 2 anchovy fillets –3 cals
- 15g (1 tbsp) baby cornichons, –8 cals
- 1 tbsp baby capers, drained –5 cals
- 1 garlic clove –2 cals
- 1 tsp Dijon mustard –4 cals
- 2 tbsp white wine vinegar –3 cals
- ½ lemon, juiced –3 cals
- 2 tbsp fresh parsley, chopped –2 cals
- 2 tbsp fresh basil, chopped –2 cals1
- 2 tbsp fresh mint, chopped –3 cals
- 2 tsp extra virgin olive oil - 45 cals
- 200g (7 oz) sustainably-caught sea bass fillets –100 cals
- 170g (6 oz) new potatoes (Charlotte or Yukon gold) –65 cals
- 2 sprays Frylight olive oil spray –1 cal
- pinch ground black pepper and sea (kosher) salt

Directions

Cut the potatoes (skin on) into half. Put into a saucepan with cold water and a pinch of salt and bring to the boil. Simmer for 15-20 mins until tender.

Rinse the anchovy fillets and capers really well and pat dry. In a mini-food processor*, add the capers, cornichons, garlic clove and anchovy fillets and pulse until finely chopped. Add the mustard, lemon juice, white wine vinegar and olive oil, and whizz again. Finally, add the fresh herbs and a good pinch of black pepper. Lightly pulse the processor again to combine well. Taste and adjust the seasoning, as required.

* If you do not have a mini-food processor, chop the herbs, vegetables and anchovy fillets as finely as you can with a small, sharp knife. Transfer to a bowl and mix in the mustard, lemon juice, white wine vinegar and olive oil, before seasoning to taste. Salsa Verde is a rustic sauce, so it will not matter if you do not have a mini-food processor to make the sauce, it will just take a little longer to make.

Heat a non-stick sauté pan over a medium heat and spritz with 2 sprays of Frylight olive oil spray. Season the flesh of the Sea Bass fillets with black pepper, then transfer to the sauté pan skin-side down for and cook for 2 minutes until the skin is crispy. Flip the fillets over, turn the heat off and cook for 1 minute more with just the heat of the pan.

Drain the potatoes and divide between 2 warm dinner plates. Spoon the salsa onto the plates beside the potatoes and then top with the cooked sea bass fillets and serve.

Serves: 2　　Ready In: 25 mins　　　　Per Serving: 246 Calories

Turkey Pot Pie

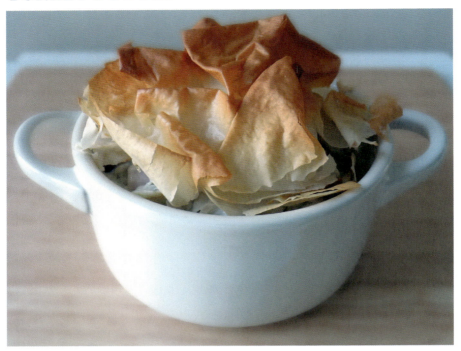

Ingredients with cals per serving

- 150g (5 oz) skinless turkey breast – 75 cals
- 1 medium stick celery (30g) –2 cals
- 1 medium leek (175g) –24 cals
- 100g (1 cup) chestnut (baby portabella) mushrooms –8 cals
- 1 medium carrot (60g) –12 cals
- 1 medium shallot (40g) –5 cals
- 1 rasher rindless back (canadian) bacon –17 cals
- 2 sheets filo pastry (c 86g/3 oz) –65 cals
- 1 tsp cornflour/corn starch –5 cals
- 25g (2 scant tbsp) 3% fat soft cheese – 14 cals
- 1 tbsp half fat crème fraîche –14 cals
- 4 sprays Frylight olive oil spray –2 cals
- 1 garlic clove –2 cals
- ½ chicken stock cube –8 cals
- ½ tsp dried mixed herbs –1 cal
- pinch ground black pepper
- pinch sea (kosher) salt

Directions

Preheat the oven to 180C fan, 375F, Gas Mark 6.

Dice the shallot, carrot and celery. Heat a non-stick sauté pan over a medium heat and spritz with 2 sprays of Frylight olive oil spray. Sauté the shallot, carrot and celery until the shallots have turned translucent. Slice the leek and mushrooms and add to the pan, continue to sauté for 4 mins until leek and mushroom are lightly cooked. Slice the turkey breast into bite size pieces and add to the pan to sauté. Mince the garlic and chop up the bacon and add to the pan to sauté.

In a small bowl, stir together the soft cheese, crème fraîche and Cornflour (corn starch) until all lumps are removed. Dissolve the ½ chicken stock cube in 80ml ($^1/_3$ cup) of boiling water. Add to the non-stick sauté pan, stirring constantly and bring to the boil until the sauce has thickened. Add the dried herbs and season to taste with salt and pepper. Divide the mixture between 2 individual pie dishes or large ramekins.

Cut the filo pastry sheets into 4 and scrunch up 4 portions on top of each pie dish. Spritz each pie with 1 spray of Frylight olive oil spray. Place on an oven tray and bake in the oven for 20-25 mins until pastry is golden.

Want to Add Potatoes? 225g (3 cups) of steamed new potatoes divided between two people adds 86 calories per portion

Serves: 2   Ready In: 35 mins   Per Serving: 254 Calories

A note from the author

Your Feedback

Thank you for choosing my Cookbook. I would love to know what you think of the recipes in this book, are any particular favourites? I would be most grateful you were able to leave a book review on the website that you purchased it from.

Further Two-Day 5:2 Diet Books

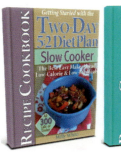 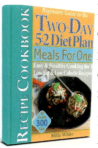

If you have enjoyed the recipes in this cookbook, you may also be interested in further books in this series:

Getting Started on The Two-Day 5:2 Diet Plan & Slow Cooker Recipe Cookbook

Beginner's Guide to the Two-Day 5:2 Diet Plan & Meals For One Recipe Cookbook.

Your Bonus 5:2 Diet Plan FREE Giveaway

As a special Thank You to my readers, I have available an exclusive & free special bonus. Sign up for my Readers Group Newsletter and receive a FREE copy of the Two-Day 5:2 Diet Plan Fast Diet Snacks Recipe Booklet.

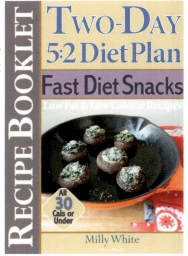

To receive your free PDF copy of this booklet, you just need to visit http://goo.gl/SciWTU and let me know where to email it to.

Let's Stay Connected

Please do also take a look at my author blog:

www.MillyWhiteCooks.com

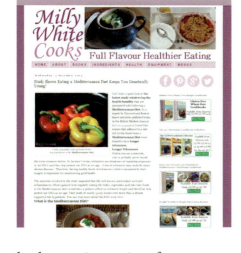

As well as details on my full range of cookbooks, you will also find articles and information on:

- Ingredients
- Cooking Techniques
- Equipment
- Health News
- Nutrition Information
- Special Offers

Every month I share a new menu of the month, showcasing recipes from my selection. You can also find me on social media too:

- MillyWhiteCooks.com
- facebook.com/MillyWhiteCooks
- instagram.com/MillyWhiteCooks
- pinterest.com/MillyWhiteCooks
- plus.google.com/+MillywhitecooksBooks/posts
- twitter.com/MillyWhiteCooks

Index

5
5:2 Nutty Maple Granola (V) — 17

A
Aromatic Duck with Plum Sauce & Sautéed Cabbage — 42

B
Baked Eggs with Roasted Asparagus & Parma Ham — 32
Banana & Walnut TeaBread (V) — 18
Beans, Lentils & Dried Peas
    Black Bean Pepper Hash (V) — 36
    Courgette & Chickpea Balti (V) — 34
    Individual Cottage Pies (V) — 48
    Ragout of Lamb & Beans — 40
Black Bean Pepper Hash (V) — 36
Breakfast Bars (V) — 19

C
Cauliflower Gratin (V) — 28
Cheesy Baked Eggs Florentine (V) — 20
Chicken & Turkey
    Chicken Veronique Lettuce Cups — 24
    Indonesian Chicken with Asian Slaw — 38
    Parma-Wrapped Chicken & Garlicky Roast Potatoes — 50
    Sweet & Sour Chicken — 35
    Tandoori Chicken Kebabs — 39
    Turkey Pot Pie — 54
Chicken Veronique Lettuce Cups — 24
Choucroute Garni with Mustard Cream Sauce — 46
Cinnamon Apple Pie Pancakes (V) — 22
Courgette & Chickpea Balti (V) — 34
Creamy Peppered Mushrooms on Toast (V) — 14
Crunchy Sesame Duck & Orange Salad — 24

D
Duck
    Aromatic Duck with Plum Sauce & Sautéed Cabbage — 42
    Crunchy Sesame Duck & Orange Salad — 24

E
Eggs
    Baked Eggs With Roasted Asparagus & Parma Ham — 32
    Cheesy Baked Eggs Florentine (V) — 20
    Cinnamon Apple Pie Pancakes (V) — 22
    Full English Breakfast Frittata — 21
    Red Pepper & Cottage Cheese Frittatas (V) — 27

F
fish & seafood
    Tuna 'Mayo' Sandwich — 29
Fish & Seafood
    Garlic & Herb Roasted Cod with Fennel En Papillote — 37
    Smoked Mackerel Pâté — 29
    Sweet Chilli Prawn Stir Fry — 31
    Tuna 'Mayo' Sandwich — 29
Full English Breakfast Frittata — 21

G
Garlic & Herb Roasted Cod with Fennel En Papillote — 37
Grilled Ruben Sandwich — 31

H
Hashed Brown Potato Cake with Mushroom & Tomato (V) — 16

I
Individual Cottage Pies (V) — 48
Indonesian Chicken with Asian Slaw — 38

L
Lamb
    Ragout of Lamb & Beans — 40

M

Mediterranean Cous Cous Salad (V) 33
Mushroom Stroganoff with Basmati Rice (V) 44

N

New Yorker Deli Breakfast Slice 15

P

Parma-Wrapped Chicken & Garlicky Roast Potatoes 50
Peach Parfait Smoothie (V) 18

R

Ragout of Lamb & Beans 40
Red Pepper & Cottage Cheese Frittatas (V) 27
Red Pepper & Roasted Garlic Humous with Crudités (V) 26

S

Salad
  Chicken Veronique Lettuce Cups 24
  Crunchy Sesame Duck & Orange Salad 24
Sausages
  Choucroute Garni with Mustard Cream Sauce 46
Smoked Mackerel Pâté 29
Spicy Roasted Vegetables and Humous Pitta (V) 30
Stuffed Peppers Provençale 23
SuperBlue Smoothie (V) 15
Superfood Soup (V) 25
Sweet & Sour Chicken 35
Sweet Chilli Prawn Stir Fry 31

T

Tandoori Chicken Kebabs 39
Tuna 'Mayo' Sandwich 29
Tuna Niçoise Salad 47
Turkey Pot Pie 54

Printed in Great Britain
by Amazon

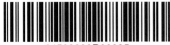